Veterinary Hematology
Atlas of Common Domestic Species

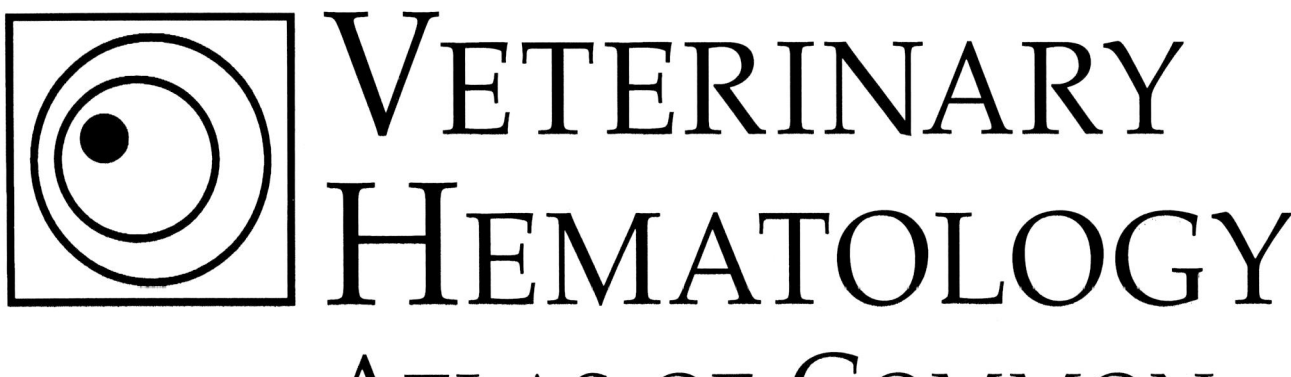

VETERINARY HEMATOLOGY
ATLAS OF COMMON DOMESTIC SPECIES

William J. Reagan

Teresa G. Sanders

Dennis B. DeNicola

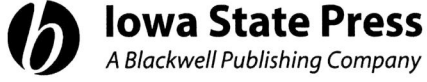 **Iowa State Press**
A Blackwell Publishing Company

WILLIAM J. REAGAN received his DVM degree from the College of Veterinary Medicine, Ohio State University, Columbus, and his PhD degree from the College of Veterinary Medicine and Biomedical Sciences, Colorado State University, Fort Collins. He is a Diplomate of the American College of Veterinary Pathologists. Dr. Reagan was formerly an Associate Professor of Veterinary Clinical Pathology, Purdue University School of Veterinary Medicine, West Lafayette, Indiana, and is currently a Research Scientist at Heska Corporation, Fort Collins, Colorado.

TERESA G. SANDERS received her Bachelor of Science degree in Medical Technology from Indiana University, Bloomington, and is presently a Clinical Pathology Laboratory Supervisor, Purdue University School of Veterinary Medicine, West Lafayette, Indiana.

DENNIS B. DeNICOLA received his DVM degree from the School of Veterinary Medicine, Purdue University, West Lafayette, Indiana, and his PhD degree from Purdue University. He is a Professor of Veterinary Clinical Pathology, Purdue University, and a Diplomate of the American College of Veterinary Pathologists.

Iowa State Press
2121 State Avenue, Ames, Iowa 50014

Orders: 1-800-862-6657   Office: 1-515-292-0140   Fax: 1-515-292-3348
www.iowastatepress.com

⊗ Printed on acid-free paper in the United States of America

First edition, 1998

Library of Congress Cataloging-in-Publication Data
Reagan, William J.
Veterinary hematology : atlas of common domestic species /
William J. Reagan, Teresa G. Sanders, Dennis B. DeNicola.—1st ed.
p.   cm.
Includes bibliographical references and index.
ISBN 0-8138-2664-0
1. Veterinary hematology—Atlases.   I. Sanders, Teresa G.
II. DeNicola, D. B.   III. Title.
SF769.5.R43   1998
636.089′615—dc21

97–7678

Last digit is the print number: 9 8 7 6 5

CONTENTS

PREFACE

The purpose of this book is to provide the fundamentals for recognizing the normal and abnormal morphological features of blood cells of the common domestic species including dogs, cats, horses, ruminants, and llamas. To accomplish this, photomicrographs that show many of the common, as well as some of the less common, blood abnormalities seen in domestic species are presented, accompanied by short morphological descriptions. A high proportion of the photomicrographs is of canine blood smears, but many of the abnormalities shown occur in other species as well. Those that are unique to one species are mentioned. Attempts were made to be as complete as possible, but, clearly, not all abnormalities that can be found in the blood are shown. There is a list of selected references that may be helpful to evaluate a morphological feature that is not described in this book. Throughout the book, in addition to the morphological features of the blood cells, some of the more common diseases or pathophysiological states in which these abnormalities may occur are mentioned. These lists of disease states are not always totally inclusive of all possible states in which these abnormalities may occur, and the readers are again referred to more-complete treatises of hematology in the references.

Wright's stain was used on the majority of blood smears that were photographed. If another stain was used, it is stated in the figure legend. If no stain is mentioned in the figure legend, the stain used was Wright's. The color reproductions of the cells were kept as consistent and as accurate as possible. The descriptions in the text and figure legends highlight these characteristics. However, depending on the exact type of stain used by the reader, the color of blood cells may be slightly different from those described in the text. Some of the major differences in staining are described in Chapter 10, Miscellaneous Findings.

The microscope objective that was used to take the photomicrographs is also listed in the figure legend. The objective is listed instead of the total original magnification in an attempt to make it easier to understand how a cell, inclusion, etc. would appear on the reader's microscope. The final magnification of all the figures is similar so that figures with the same objective listed can be compared directly.

This textbook should be useful to the novice and experienced hematologist alike. The glossary, which defines many of the terms used in the text, may be more useful to the novice. Two appendixes, which present methods used in the Purdue University Veterinary Teaching Hospital Clinical Pathology Laboratory for semiquantitation of some of the morphological abnormalities, may be useful to the novice as well as the experienced hematologist. These appendixes should be helpful guidelines for reproducibly recording morphological abnormalities that may be present in a blood smear.

Finally, we have many people to thank for their assistance in developing this atlas. First and most important are our families, who provided us with the time and support to pursue this project. Special thanks go to Julie Clements-Reagan for her contribution to the graphic design of the book and to Colleen Sherman for her word processing support. We also thank the technicians and clinical pathology residents of the Purdue University Veterinary Teaching Hospital Clinical Pathology Laboratory for suggestions on content, as well as help in acquiring the case material used in the book. Some additional material was obtained from glass slides that were submitted to the American Society of Veterinary Clinical Pathology (ASVCP) annual slide review; those slides are identified in the legends. We thank the society and contributors for this material. Finally, we appreciate the support and opportunity that Iowa State University Press has given us to develop this resource.

VETERINARY HEMATOLOGY
ATLAS OF COMMON DOMESTIC SPECIES

CHAPTER ONE

HEMATOPOIESIS

GENERAL FEATURES

All blood cells have a finite life span, but in normal animals the numbers of cells in circulation are maintained at a fairly constant level. To accomplish this, cells in circulation need to be constantly replenished, and this occurs by the production and release of cells from the bone marrow. Production sites in the bone marrow are commonly referred to as medullary sites. In times of increased demand, production can also occur outside the bone marrow in sites such as spleen, liver, and lymph nodes. These sites are called extramedullary sites.

Hematopoiesis, the production of blood cells, is a complex and highly regulated process. All blood cells in the bone marrow arise from a common stem cell. This pluripotent stem cell gives rise to several stages of committed progenitor cells, which then differentiate into cells of the erythrocytic, granulocytic, megakaryocytic, and agranulocytic (monocytic and lymphocytic) lineages. The end result of this development process is the release of red blood cells, white blood cells, and platelets into the circulation. At the light microscopic level, it is impossible to accurately identify the early stem cells in the bone marrow, but the more differentiated stages of development can be identified and are graphically depicted in Figure 1.1 and described on the following pages.

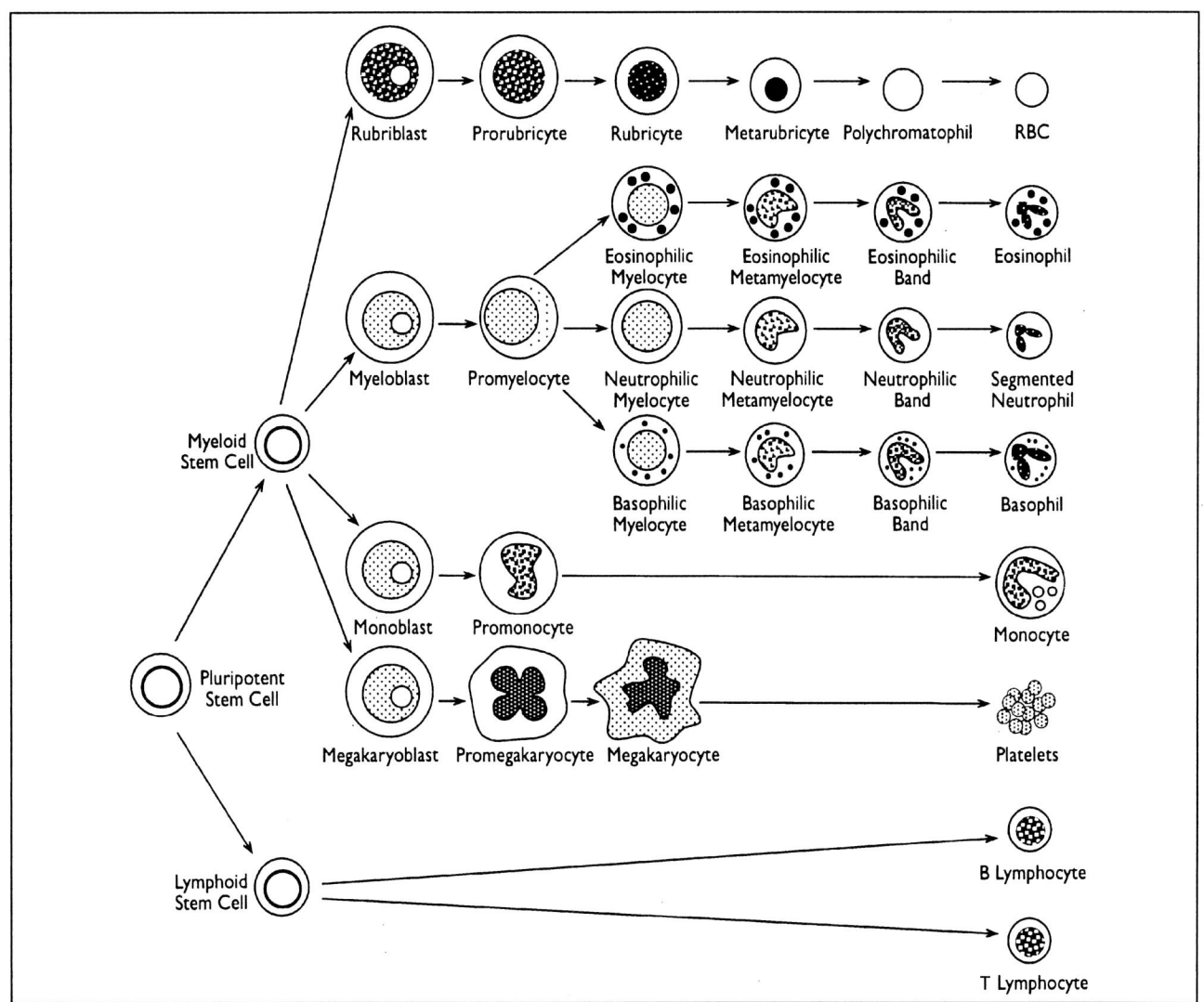

Figure 1.1. Overview of hematopoiesis.

3

Figure 1.2 shows a histological section of a bone marrow core biopsy from a dog. Note that there is a mixture of approximately 50% hematopoietic cells and 50% fat that is surrounded by bony trabeculae. The specific types of bone marrow cells can be difficult to recognize in histological sections at this low-power magnification, but the very large cells present are megakaryocytes. Cells are easier to identify on a smear from a bone marrow aspirate (Figure 1.3). The cells that are present include erythrocytic and granulocytic precursors, and a megakaryocyte. To classify these three different cell types, there are some general

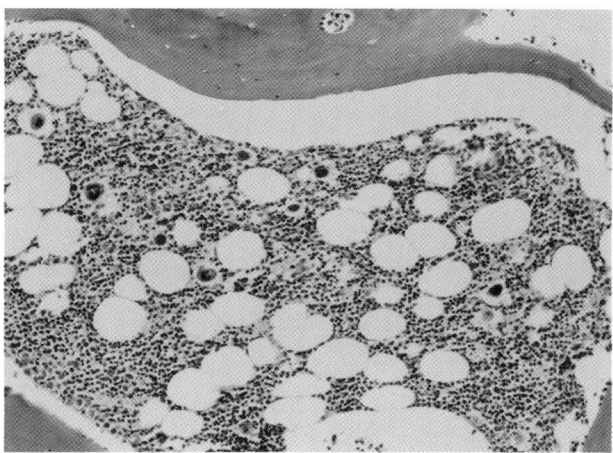

Figure 1.2. Histological section of canine bone marrow. Pink bony trabeculae are present in the lower left corner, lower right corner, and top of the photomicrograph and surround the hematopoietic cells and fat. The fat is the round to oval, clear areas. The erythrocytic and granulocytic precursor cells are the many small, round purple structures. The larger, densely staining purple structures distributed throughout the marrow space are megakaryocytes. Canine bone marrow core biopsy; hematoxylin and eosin stain; 10× objective.

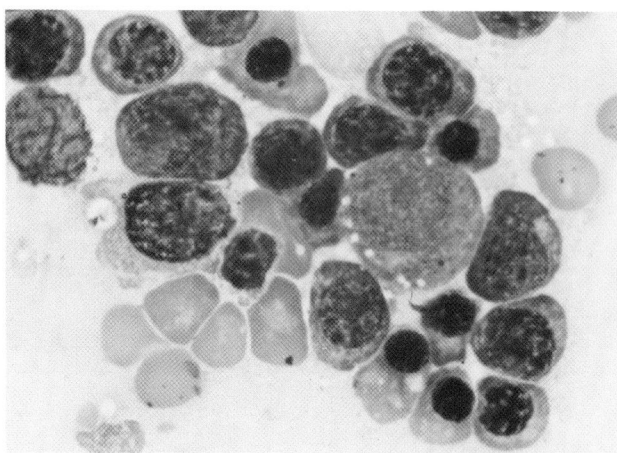

Figure 1.4. Erythrocytic precursors. The majority of the intact cells present are early erythrocytic precursors with centrally located round nuclei and deep blue cytoplasm. The cells with round eccentrically placed nuclei and reddish-blue cytoplasm are late-stage erythrocytic precursors. The largest cell in the right center of the field that has small pink granules in the cytoplasm is a promyelocyte. Canine bone marrow smear; 100× objective.

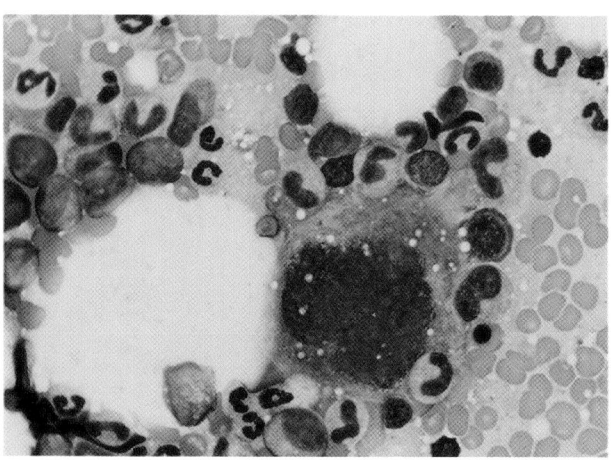

Figure 1.3. Megakaryocyte, erythrocytic precursors, and granulocytic precursors. The megakaryocyte is the largest cell located in right center of the field. The early erythrocytic precursors have central round nuclei and deep blue cytoplasm. The early granulocytic precursors have oval to indented nuclei and blue cytoplasm. There is a granulocytic predominance in this field. Canine bone marrow smear; 50× objective.

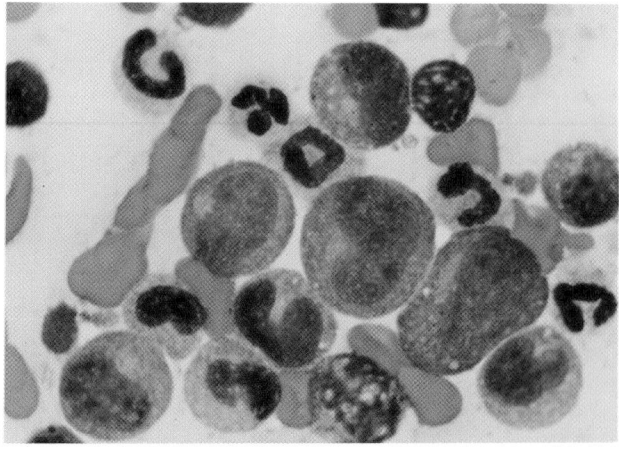

Figure 1.5. Granulocytic precursors. The majority of the intact cells present are granulocytic precursors with oval to indented nuclei and blue cytoplasm. The larger immature forms have small, pink cytoplasmic granules. The cytoplasm becomes less blue as the cells mature. Canine bone marrow smear; 100× objective.

features that can be used. Megakaryocytes are easy to distinguish by their very large size; the majority of them are 100 to 200 μm in diameter compared to approximately 20 to 30 μm for the largest granulocytic or erythrocytic precursors.

Cells of the erythrocytic lineage can be initially distinguished from those of the granulocytic lineage based upon nuclear shape and color of cytoplasm (Figures 1.4 and 1.5). Cells of the erythrocytic lineage have very round nuclei throughout most stages of development. In contrast, the nuclei of cells of the granulocytic lineage become indented and segmented as they mature. In addition, the cytoplasm of early erythrocytic precursors is much bluer than that of the granulocytic precursors.

There are several additional common morphological features that occur during development of both erythrocytic and granulocytic precursors. Both cell and nucleus decrease in size as they mature. As cells lose their capacity to divide, there is a loss of nucleoli and a condensation of nuclear chromatin. Changes in the cytoplasm are also occurring. As the hemoglobin content in erythrocytic precursors increases, the cytoplasm becomes less blue and more red. As maturation proceeds in the granulocytic cells, the cytoplasm also becomes less blue.

ERYTHROPOIESIS

There are several stages of erythrocyte development that are recognizable in the bone marrow. Figure 1.6

depicts erythrocyte development and Plate 1 shows the morphology of all erythrocytic precursors. Briefly, erythrocyte development is as follows.

The rubriblast is the first morphologically recognizable erythrocytic precursor. The rubriblast is a large round cell with a large round nucleus with coarsely granular chromatin and a prominent nucleolus. These cells have small amounts of deep blue cytoplasm. The rubriblast divides to produce two prorubricytes.

The prorubricyte is round and of equal size or sometimes larger than the rubriblast. The nucleus is round with a coarsely granular chromatin pattern. A nucleolus is typically not present. There is a small amount of deep blue cytoplasm, often with a prominent perinuclear clear zone. Each prorubricyte divides to form two rubricytes.

The rubricyte is smaller than the prorubricyte. The nucleus is still round, and the coarsely granular chromatin is more condensed compared to the earlier stages. There is a small amount of deep blue cytoplasm, although some of the more mature rubricytes have reddish-blue cytoplasm. At the rubricyte stage, there are two divisions; the rubricytes then mature into metarubricytes.

The metarubricyte is smaller than the rubricyte. The nucleus is round to slightly oval, is centrally to eccentrically located, and has very condensed chromatin. There is a moderate amount of blue to reddish-blue cytoplasm. From the metarubricyte stage on, there is no further division of the cells, just maturation.

The highly condensed pyknotic nucleus of the

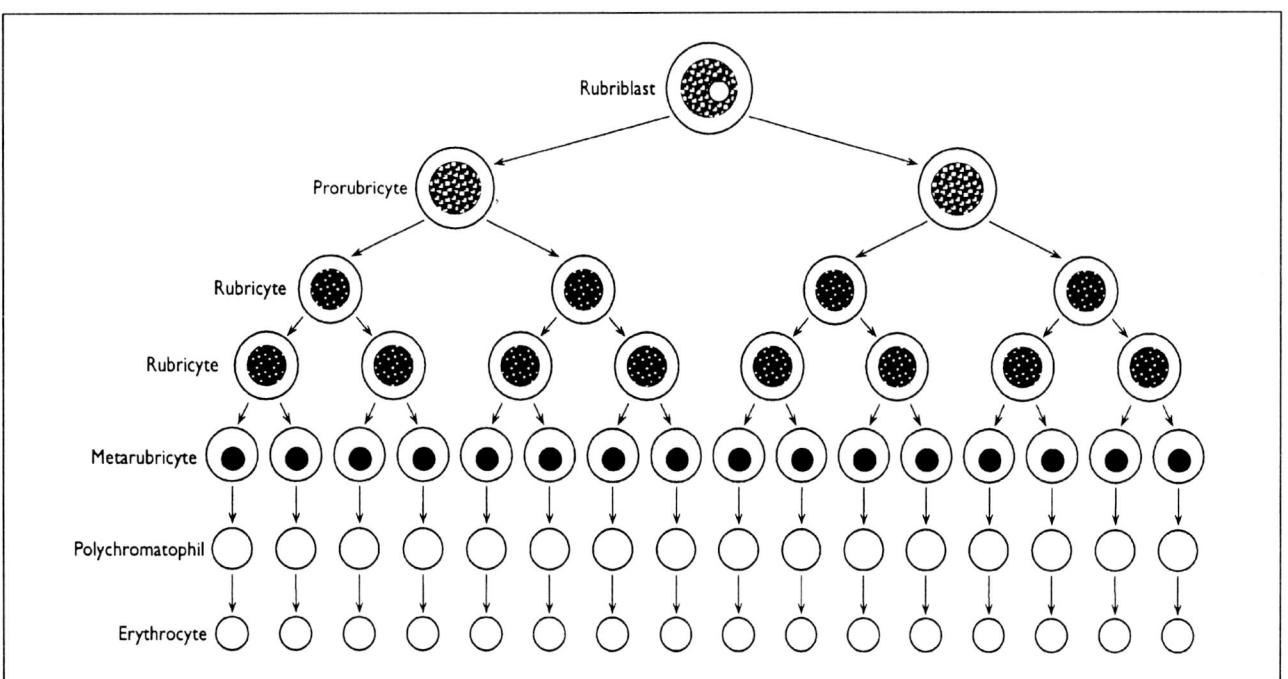

Figure 1.6. Overview of erythropoiesis.

metarubricyte is extruded from the cell, and this cell becomes a polychromatophil. Polychromatophils are round cells without a nucleus and have bluish cytoplasm. As a polychromatophil matures, it becomes less blue and more red to become a mature red blood cell. The mature red blood cells have species-dependent morphological features, which are described in Chapter 2.

GRANULOPOIESIS

Granulopoiesis is depicted in Figure 1.7 and Plate 2. In the bone marrow, there are three types of granulocytes, which include cells of the neutrophilic, eosinophilic, and basophilic lineages. Cells of the neutrophilic lineage are the predominant type of granulocyte present, and their development is described first.

The myeloblast is the first recognizable granulocytic precursor in the bone marrow. It is a large cell with a round to oval nucleus with a finely granular chromatin pattern and one or more prominent nucleoli. The amount of cytoplasm is small to moderate and blue. Each myeloblast divides to form two promyelocytes. Promyelocytes look similar to myeloblasts except they may not have nucleoli, and they may have a perinuclear clear zone within the cytoplasm. The distinguishing feature of promyelocytes is that they contain multiple, very small pink to purple granules in the cytoplasm; these are known as primary granules.

Promyelocytes divide to produce myelocytes.

The myelocyte is smaller than the earlier precursors and has a round to oval to slightly indented nucleus with finely to moderately granular chromatin. These cells have moderate amounts of blue cytoplasm. At this stage, primary granules are no longer being produced, and now secondary granules are formed. These secondary granules are larger than the primary granules.

In neutrophilic myelocytes, the secondary granules are light pink and are very difficult to recognize with the light microscope. The myelocyte goes through two divisions, and the resulting progeny mature into metamyelocytes. From the metamyelocyte stage forward, the cells no longer divide.

The metamyelocyte is smaller than the myelocyte and has a kidney-shaped nucleus. The chromatin is moderately granular and more condensed and clumped than that in the myelocyte. The cytoplasm is blue and contains primary and secondary granules. Both types of granules in the metamyelocyte, and subsequent stages of development are not easily seen light microscopically. Metamyelocytes develop into band neutrophils. Band neutrophils are round and smaller than metamyelocytes, have horseshoe-shaped nuclei, and have moderate amounts of blue to light blue cytoplasm. The band neutrophil will mature into a segmented neutrophil, which is a small cell with faintly blue to pink cytoplasm and a segmented nu-

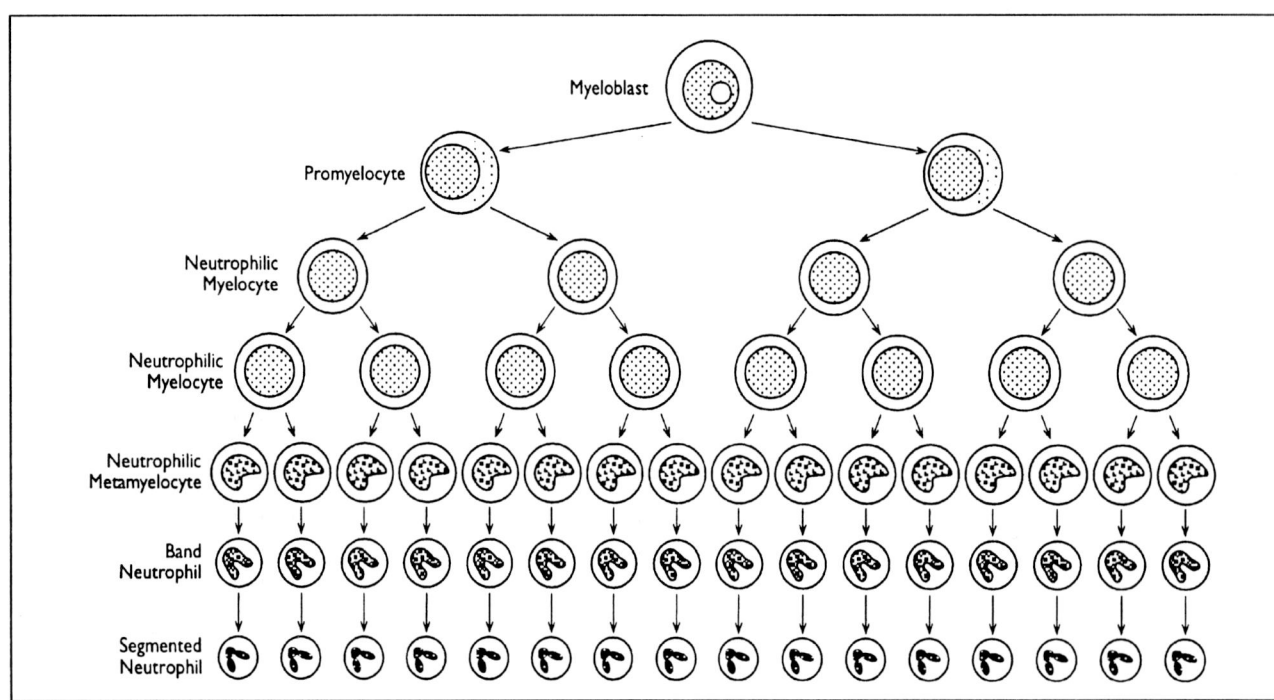

Figure 1.7. Overview of neutrophilic granulopoiesis.

cleus. The nuclear chromatin is coarsely granular and clumped.

Mature eosinophils and basophils and their precursors are found in very low numbers in the normal bone marrow. The production of these cells is very similar to that of neutrophils and only major differences are described below (Figure 1.1). The development is identical until the myelocytic stage, which is when eosinophilic and basophilic myelocytes can be distinguished from neutrophilic myelocytes by the color of the secondary granules. The eosinophilic and basophilic myelocytes contain reddish to reddish-orange and purple secondary granules respectively. Eosinophilic and basophilic metamyelocytes and bands can also be recognized by the presence of the unique secondary granules.

The last stage of development is the mature eosinophil and basophil. The eosinophil is often slightly larger than the mature neutrophil, and the nucleus is not as tightly segmented. The cytoplasm contains reddish to reddish-orange granules. The mature basophil is a round cell that is slightly larger than the neutrophil, with a segmented nucleus with condensed chromatin. The cytoplasm is light purple and may contain granules. There are some unique species-dependent features of mature eosinophils and basophils, which are described in Chapter 5.

MONOCYTOPOIESIS

The precursors of monocytes arise from committed stem cells, which are common precursors for both cells of the granulocytic and monocytic lineage. Monocyte development is depicted in Figure 1.1. In normal bone marrow, very few cells of the monocytic lineage are present. Monoblasts are the first microscopically recognizable precursors in bone marrow, although they can be impossible to differentiate from myeloblasts. Monoblasts give rise to promonocytes. A promonocyte is a large cell with an oval to sometimes indented nucleus with a reticular (net-like) or lacy chromatin pattern. These cells have small to moderate amounts of blue cytoplasm and can be difficult to distinguish from neutrophilic myelocytes or metamyelocytes. Promonocytes give rise to monocytes, which are larger than segmented neutrophils. The nucleus of the monocyte has multiple indentations. The nuclear chromatin has areas of condensation but has a lacy or reticular pattern compared to the condensed chromatin pattern of the mature neutrophil. The cytoplasm is moderate in amount and is typically blue-gray, often with discrete multiple vacuoles.

MEGAKARYOCYTOPOIESIS AND PLATELET PRODUCTION

Megakaryocytopoiesis is quite unique compared to the development of the other blood cells and is depicted in Figure 1.1. The megakaryoblasts are the first morphologically recognizable precursors of the megakaryocytic lineage in bone marrow, but can be impossible to differentiate from other blast cells. The megakaryoblast is a large cell with a single round nucleus and prominent nucleolus. This cell differentiates into a promegakaryocyte, which is larger than the megakaryoblast and has a multilobed nucleus with dark blue agranular cytoplasm. The promegakaryocyte gives rise to the megakaryocyte (Figure 1.8), which is easily recognized in the bone marrow due to its large size (typically 100 to 200 μm). This large cell has a large multilobulated nucleus and abundant granular cytoplasm.

Platelets are formed from the cytoplasm of megakaryocytes by the formation of a structure known as a proplatelet. The proplatelet is fragmented into multiple platelets. The resulting platelets are discoid-shaped small cells that do not have nuclei and have light pink cytoplasm with sometimes distinct purple granules.

LYMPHOPOIESIS

Lymphocytes arise from the same common stem cell precursor as do the other bone marrow cells (Figure 1.1). Multiple stages of differentiation of lymphocytes

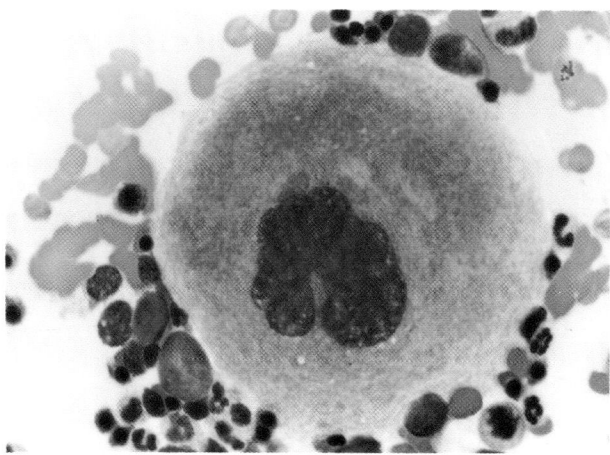

Figure 1.8. Megakaryocyte. The megakaryocyte is the large cell in the center with a multilobulated irregular nuclei and abundant granular cytoplasm. Canine bone marrow smear; 50× objective.

in bone marrow cannot be recognized light microscopically, but there are two main types of lymphocytes found in the peripheral blood: B and T lymphocytes. These two cell types look similar and cannot be differentiated based on morphology alone, but their functions are quite different. In bone marrow, low numbers of small lymphocytes and rare medium and large lymphocytes are present (Figure 1.9). The exact

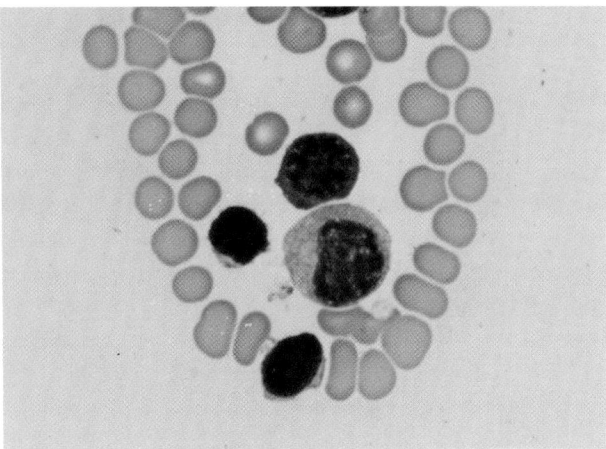

Figure 1.9. Lymphocytes. The two smallest round cells (left center) that are slightly larger than red blood cells, with round to oval nuclei and small amounts of light blue cytoplasm, are small lymphocytes. The largest cell in the center is a neutrophilic granulocytic precursor. The round cell (above the granulocytic precursor) with a round nucleus, very condensed chromatin, and a rim of deep blue cytoplasm is a rubricyte. Feline bone marrow smear; 100× objective.

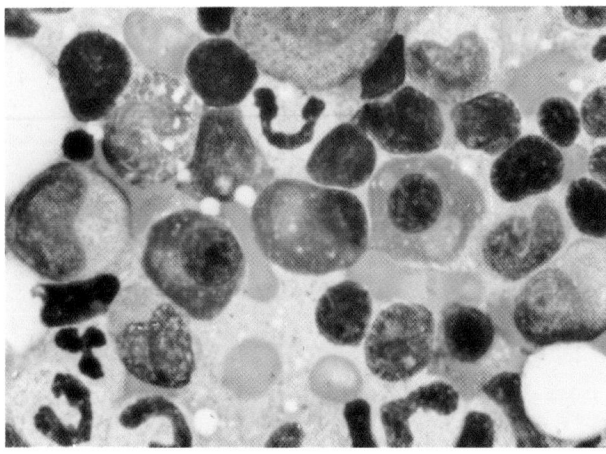

Figure 1.10. Plasma cells. The three cells (center) with eccentrically placed round nuclei, with coarse clumped chromatin, and a moderate amount of deep blue cytoplasm with perinuclear clear zones are plasma cells. The other cells are mainly granulocytic precursors. Canine bone marrow smear; 100× objective.

number of lymphocytes present in bone marrow is species dependent.

The small lymphocyte is a small round cell with a round to slightly indented nucleus. In some areas the nuclear chromatin has a very smooth glassy appearance, and in other areas it is more clumped or smudged. Overall, the chromatin is not as condensed as that of a rubricyte, which is the cell type with which it is most often confused. The lymphocyte has a small amount of light blue cytoplasm. The medium and large lymphocyte, as the names imply, are larger than the small lymphocyte. The nuclei are round and the chromatin is finely granular with some areas of condensation. The nucleus of the large lymphocyte typically has a nucleolus and is known as a lymphoblast. Both cell types have small amounts of light to moderate blue cytoplasm.

In addition to lymphocytes, low numbers of plasma cells can be seen in bone marrow (Figure 1.10). These cells are the end stage of differentiation of B lymphocytes and are round with eccentrically placed round nuclei. The nuclear chromatin is very condensed and clumped with clear areas between the clumps. Plasma cells have moderate amounts of deep blue cytoplasm with a prominent perinuclear clear zone.

OTHER CELLS OF THE BONE MARROW

Macrophage

Bone marrow macrophages are present in low numbers (Figure 1.11). These cells are large and have an oval to indented nucleus. The nuclear chromatin is reticular or net-like. The moderate to abundant amounts of blue cytoplasm often are very foamy and may contain multiple, variably sized vacuoles. Often within these cells there can be phagocytized debris or iron pigment, known as hemosiderin. In general, hemosiderin is not identified in normal cat bone marrow.

Osteoclast

Osteoclasts are rarely found in bone marrow smears. Osteoclasts are similar in size to megakaryocytes, and these two cell types are often confused (Figure 1.12). The osteoclast has multiple, individual round to oval nuclei. In contrast, the nucleus of the mature megakaryocyte is multilobulated. The osteoclast cytoplasm is granular and light blue to red.

Osteoblast

Osteoblasts are also found in very low numbers in normal bone marrow. The size of these cells is very similar to that of the macrophage, and the morphology is somewhat similar to that of the plasma cell, including an eccentrically placed round nucleus and prominent perinuclear clear zone (Figure 1.13). The nucleus has a granular chromatin pattern, usually with a prominent single nucleolus. The cytoplasm is a light to moderate blue. In contrast, the plasma cell is smaller in size and the nuclear chromatin is much more condensed with no prominent nucleoli.

Mast Cell

Mast cells can be found in very low numbers in bone marrow. These cells are round with a round, centrally located nucleus (Figure 1.14). These cells are easily recognized by the small purple granules that fill the cytoplasm. Often in these cells the granularity is so great that it hides the nuclei. Mast cells are often present within intact bone marrow particles.

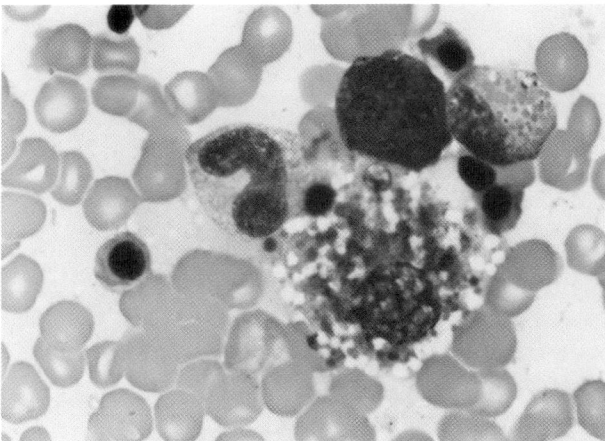

Figure 1.11. Macrophage. The large cell (right center) with abundant vacuolated cytoplasm and a round nucleus is a macrophage. The red-brown granules in the cytoplasm are consistent with hemosiderin. Canine bone marrow smear; 100× objective.

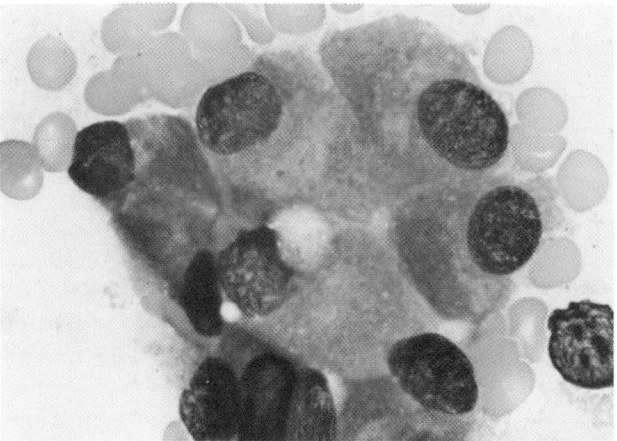

Figure 1.13. Osteoblasts. The nucleated cells with abundant blue cytoplasm (center) that form a circle are osteoblasts. These cells appear similar to plasma cells; however, they are larger than plasma cells and the nuclear chromatin patterns are less coarse. Canine bone marrow smear; 100× objective.

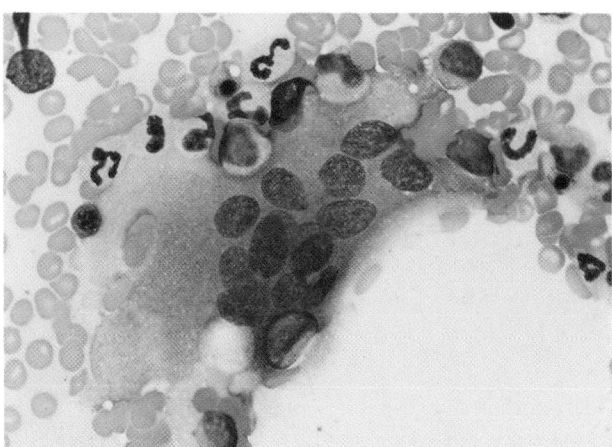

Figure 1.12. Osteoclast. The very large cell (center) with multiple, individual round to oval nuclei and granular cytoplasm is an osteoclast. The large clear area in the lower right quadrant is a large fat droplet, which is partially indenting the osteoclast. Canine bone marrow smear; 50× objective.

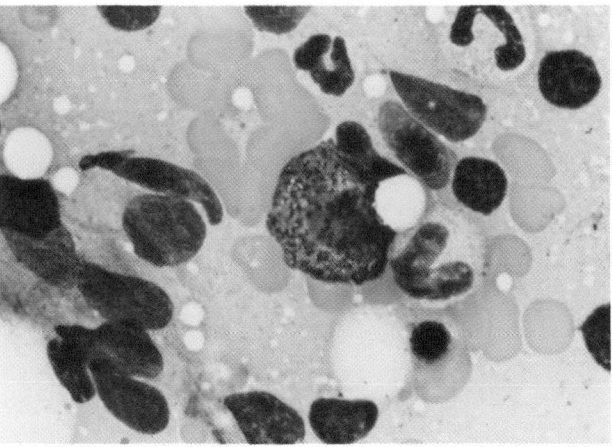

Figure 1.14. Mast cell. The cell (center) with abundant purple cytoplasmic granules is a mast cell. The granules almost obscure the round nucleus. A small fat droplet (round clear structure) is partially indenting the right side of the cell. Canine bone marrow smear; 100× objective.

PLATE 1. Red Blood Cell Development

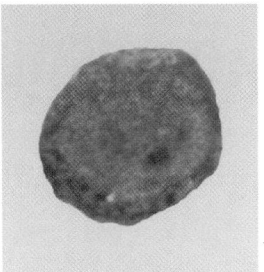

Rubriblast

The rubriblast is a large round cell with a large round nucleus, coarsely granular chromatin, and a nucleolus. This cell has small amounts of deep blue cytoplasm.

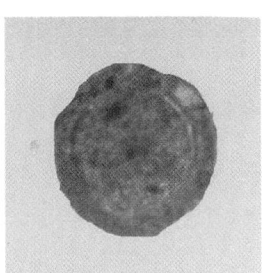

Prorubricyte

The prorubricyte is a large round cell with a round nucleus with a coarsely granular chromatin pattern. This cell typically lacks a nucleolus. There is a small amount of deep blue cytoplasm with often a prominent perinuclear clear zone.

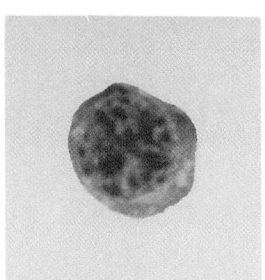

Rubricyte

The rubricyte is a round cell with a round, centrally located nucleus; it is smaller than the prorubricyte. The coarsely granular chromatin is more condensed compared with the earlier stages of development, and irregular clear areas are present between the chromatin clumps. The cytoplasm varies from deep blue to reddish-blue. Early rubricytes typically have more bluish cytoplasm, and later rubricytes stain more red as the amount of hemoglobin increases.

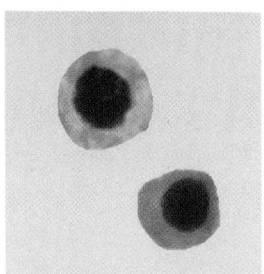

Metarubricyte

The metarubricyte is smaller than the rubricyte. The nucleus is round to oval, usually slightly eccentrically located, and has very condensed chromatin. There are small to moderate amounts of blue to reddish-blue cytoplasm. The metarubricytes, with more-reddish cytoplasm, contain more hemoglobin.

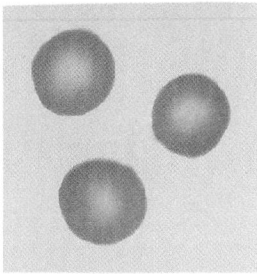

Polychromatophil

The polychromatophil does not have a nucleus, and cytoplasm is blue to reddish-blue. As polychromatophils mature, they become less blue and more red due to increased amounts of hemoglobin.

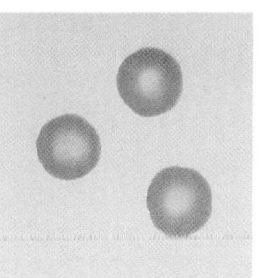

Red blood cell

The red blood cell does not have a nucleus, and the cytoplasm is reddish to reddish-orange. The central pallor present here is due to the biconcave discoid shape of the cells.

PLATE 2. White Blood Cell Development

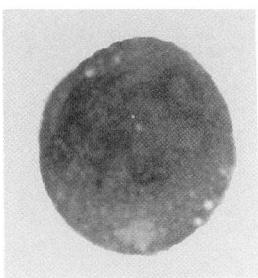

Myeloblast

The myeloblast is a large, round to oval cell with a round to oval nucleus with a finely stippled chromatin pattern and usually prominent nucleolus or multiple nucleoli. There is a small to moderate amount of blue cytoplasm and no prominent cytoplasmic granules.

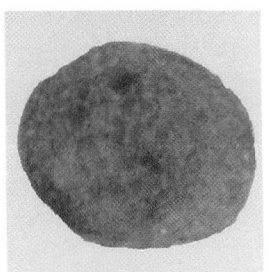

Promyelocyte

The promyelocyte is a large, round to oval cell with a round to oval nucleus. The nuclear chromatin pattern is finely granular. A nucleolus or multiple nucleoli may or may not be present. A perinuclear clear zone is often present but not shown here. The moderate amount of cytoplasm is blue and contains multiple, fine, pink to purple granules, which are primary granules.

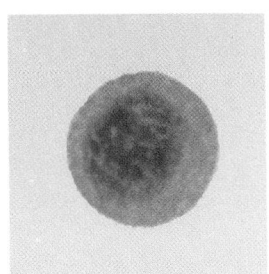

Neutrophilic myelocyte

The neutrophilic myelocyte is a round cell that is smaller than the myeloblast and the progranulocyte. The nucleus is round to oval and may contain a single indentation. The chromatin pattern is finely to moderately granular. Nucleoli are not present. The moderate amounts of blue cytoplasm contain multiple secondary granules, also called specific granules. These secondary granules are pink for the neutrophilic lineage and difficult to see. The secondary granules for the eosinophilic and basophilic lineages are generally reddish and purple respectively.

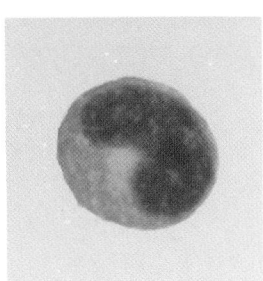

Neutrophilic metamyelocyte

The neutrophilic metamyelocyte is a round cell with a kidney-shaped nucleus. The chromatin is moderately granular and more condensed than that of the myelocyte. The moderate amounts of blue cytoplasm contain secondary granules, which are difficult to see. The secondary granules of the eosinophilic and basophilic metamyelocyte are generally reddish and purple respectively.

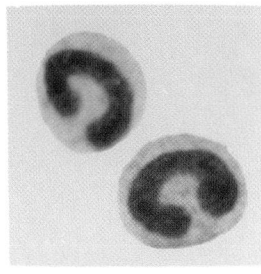

Band neutrophil

The band neutrophil is a round cell with a horseshoe-shaped nucleus. The nuclear membranes may have parallel sides, although slight indentations are acceptable. The cytoplasm is blue to light blue and contains secondary granules. These granules are difficult to see in the band neutrophil. The secondary granules of the band eosinophil and basophil are generally reddish and purple respectively.

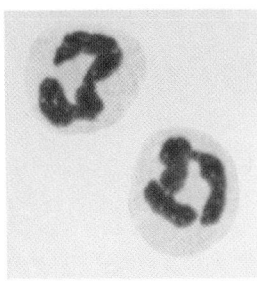

Segmented neutrophil

The segmented neutrophil is a small round cell with a single nucleus, which has multiple segmentations. The nuclear chromatin is very condensed. There is a moderate amount of light blue to pink cytoplasm.

CHAPTER TWO

NORMAL RED BLOOD CELL MORPHOLOGY

The morphological features of mature red blood cells of dogs, cats, horses, and ruminants are generally very similar in that they all lack nuclei, stain reddish to reddish-orange, and generally are biconcave discoid-shaped cells. The major differences are in the size of the red blood cells and the degree of central pallor. Listed from largest to smallest in size are dog, cat, horse, cow, sheep, and goat red blood cells. The central pallor is the lighter-staining area in the middle of the cell, due to close association of the membranes in this region (Figure 2.1). Dog red blood cells have the most-prominent central pallor. In cats, horses, and ruminants, central pallor is not prominent. In contrast to the other domestic species, normal llama red blood cells are quite different in morphology. Although they lack nuclei and stain reddish to reddish-orange, they are small elliptical discs that lack a biconcave shape and central pallor. Table 2.1 summarizes the morphological features, and Figures 2.2–2.8 show photomicrographs of normal red blood cells of the common domestic species.

Two other morphological features that may be present in normal animals are rouleaux and anisocytosis. Rouleaux are organized linear arrays of red blood cells stacked one on top of another (see Figure 3.8). This change can best be seen in thicker areas of blood smears, known as the body of the slide. Rouleaux are most prominent in normal horses, but also occur in cats and to a much lesser degree in dogs. Rouleaux formation is related to differences in charges at the red blood cell surface, and changes in these charges can result in increased degrees of rouleaux formation. With inflammatory disease, there often are increased levels of globulins in the blood that result in changes in protein charges, and thus increased rouleaux in most animals. In llamas and the bovine species, there is generally a lack of rouleaux in normal and disease states. Anisocytosis is defined as a variation in red blood cell size. Anisocytosis is mainly present in normal cats and cows (Figures 2.3 and 2.5).

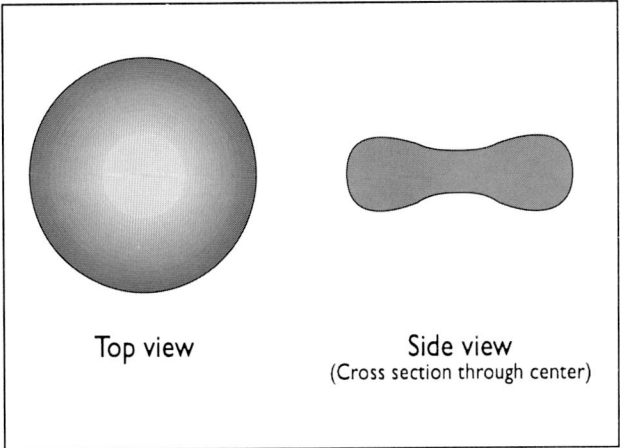

Top view

Side view
(Cross section through center)

Figure 2.1. Graphical representation of a normal dog red blood cell. Note the central zone of pallor is due to the closer apposition of membranes and a decreased amount of hemoglobin in this region.

Table 2.1
Morphological features of normal red blood cells

Animal	Diameter (μm)	Central Pallor	Rouleaux	Anisocytosis
Dog	7.0	++	+	−
Cat	5.8	+	++	+
Horse	5.7	±	+++	−
Cow	5.5	+	−	+
Sheep	4.5	+	±	±
Goat	3.2	±	±	+
Llama	4.0 × 7.0*	−	−	±

Source: Adapted from Jain, Nemi C. 1986. *Schalm's Veterinary Hematology*, 4th ed. Philadelphia: Lea & Febiger.

*Since these cells are not round, the approximate width and length of the cells are given.

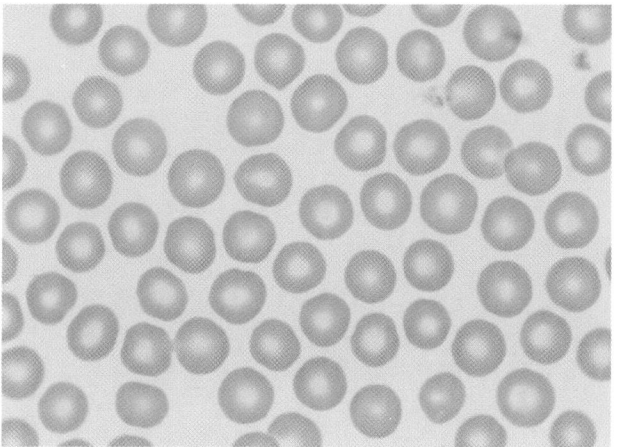

Figure 2.2. Dog red blood cells. The majority of the cells are of similar size and have prominent central pallor. Canine blood smear; 100× objective.

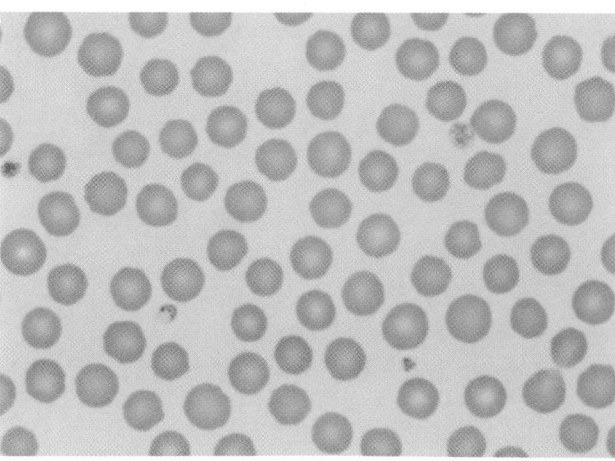

Figure 2.5. Cow red blood cells. There is slight variation in the size of these cells (anisocytosis), and they typically have limited central pallor. Bovine blood smear; 100× objective.

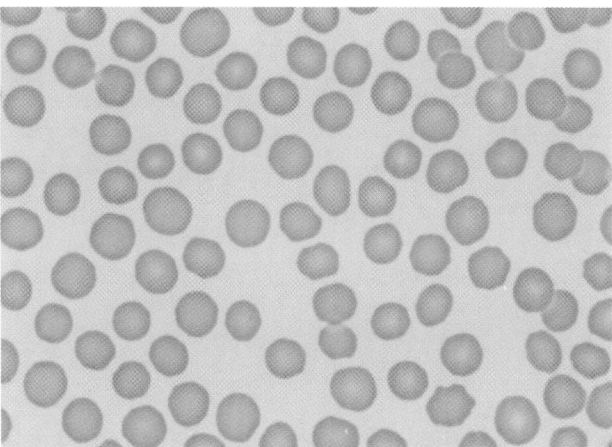

Figure 2.3. Cat red blood cells. These cells are smaller than dog red blood cells, there is slight variation in size (anisocytosis), and they have limited central pallor. Feline blood smear; 100× objective.

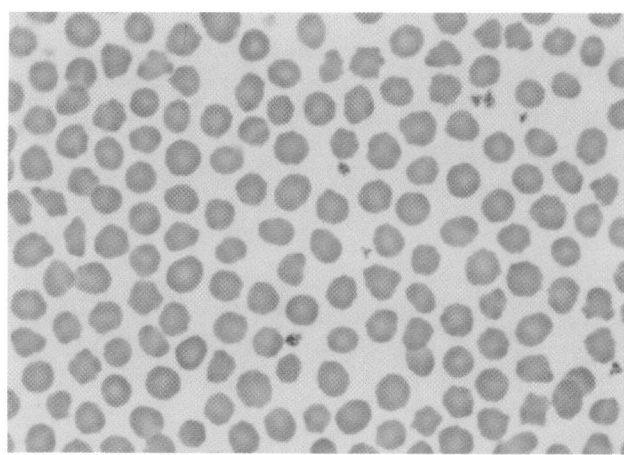

Figure 2.6. Sheep red blood cells. Note the very small size of these cells, compared with dog red blood cells, and their limited central pallor. There is also slight variation in size (anisocytosis) and shape (poikilocytosis) of these cells. Ovine blood smear; 100× objective.

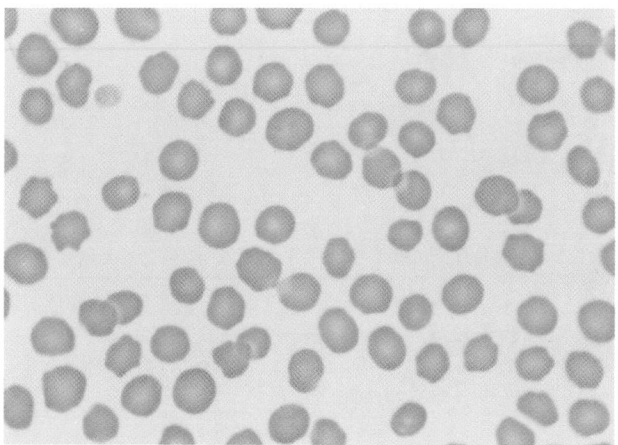

Figure 2.4. Horse red blood cells. These cells are smaller than dog red blood cells, and they have minimal central pallor. Equine blood smear; 100× objective.

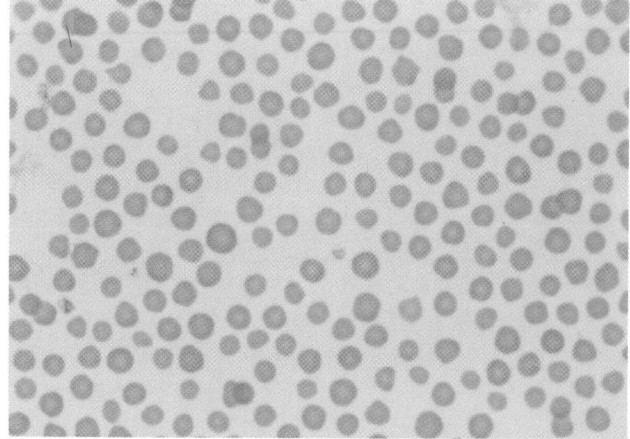

Figure 2.7. Goat red blood cells. Note the extremely small size of the cells and the minimal central pallor. It is also common to have slight variation in size (anisocytosis) and shape (poikilocytosis). Caprine blood smear; 100× objective.

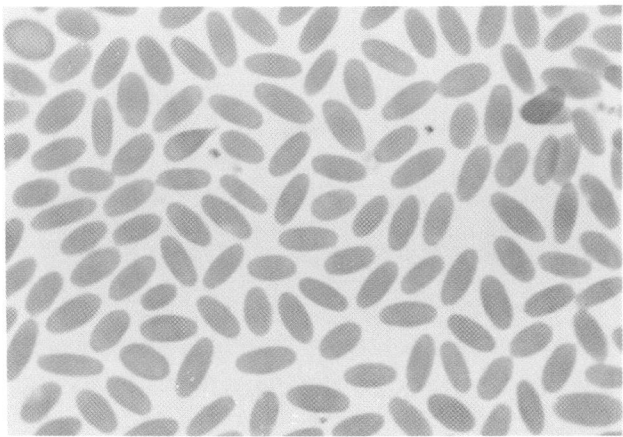

Figure 2.8. Llama red blood cells. These cells are elliptical and lack central pallor. Llama blood smear; 100× objective.

CHAPTER THREE

VARIATIONS IN RED BLOOD CELL MORPHOLOGY

Variations in the morphology of red blood cells can occur in animals with various disease and pathophysiological states. To better understand the development of these changes, they will be grouped into five categories: morphological features associated with (1) a regenerative response, (2) immune-mediated damage, (3) oxidative injury, (4) membrane/metabolic disorder, and (5) mechanical fragmentation. These categories are not mutually exclusive, and morphological features that are described in one category may be seen in multiple physiological or disease states. The more common physiological or disease states in which these cell types are seen are mentioned, but these lists are not meant to be comprehensive. These changes will often be demonstrated by photomicrographs of canine blood smears, but most of these abnormalities occur in the other species as well.

A general term that is used in describing variations in red blood cell morphology is poikilocytosis, which is defined as abnormally shaped red blood cells in circulation. If the shape change that is present can be subclassified using a more specific term, the more specific term should be used.

REGENERATIVE RESPONSE

Anemias can be classified into two major categories: nonregenerative and regenerative. A nonregenerative anemia is due to inadequate production of red blood cells by bone marrow; red blood cells that are present in circulation often appear normal. In contrast, a regenerative anemia is one in which the bone marrow has responded to a demand for red blood cells by increasing production and releasing into the circulation adequate numbers of immature red blood cells, known as polychromatophils (Figure 3.1). These cells have bluish to reddish-blue cytoplasm and are typically slightly larger than mature red blood cells. Also, due to the increased pliability of these cells, they do not always take on the classic discoid shape but may have multiple infoldings or outfoldings of the membranes and thus appear as target or bar cells, which are described next. Although polychromatophils can be identified on Wright's-stained preparations due to their bluish coloration, they can also be identified easily by staining a blood sample with new methylene blue.

In new methylene blue–stained preparations, polychromatophils are called reticulocytes (Figure 3.2), and they will stain bluish-green, as will mature red blood cells. In addition, the polychromatophils will have irregular net-like structures, known as reticulum, within the cells. The reticulum is irregular clumps of ribosomal RNA and organelles, such as mitochondria. In most species, there is only one type of reticulocyte. However, in cats there are two forms of reticulocytes: punctate and aggregate (Figure 3.3). The aggregate reticulocytes have abundant reticulum whereas punctate reticulocytes have only a few isolated dots of reticulum, which do not coalesce.

In addition to finding polychromatophils, other features that may be seen in regenerative anemias are nucleated red blood cells, basophilic stippling, anisocytosis, and Howell-Jolly bodies. It is not exactly clear why nucleated red blood cells (Figure 3.4) are found in circulation during a regenerative response. It may be that these cells are released due to mild bone marrow stromal damage or due to the increased demand for red blood cells.

When demand for red blood cells is great, production occurs in extramedullary sites such as the liver and spleen, with the subsequent potential release of nucleated red blood cells into circulation. When nucleated red blood cells are present without the presence of adequate polychromasia, underlying causes of bone marrow damage are likely. A classic example of this is animals with lead poisoning.

Basophilic stippling (Figure 3.5) can be seen on Wright's-stained smears as small, variably sized blue dots in the cytoplasm of red blood cells. In most cases, the dots are retained RNA and are most commonly seen during regenerative responses in ruminants, but they also can be seen during regeneration in other species. Basophilic stippling may be seen in lead poisoning because lead inhibits an enzyme that is important in the degradation of RNA.

Anisocytosis has been previously defined and occurs in a regenerative response, typically due to the presence of large polychromatophils.

Howell-Jolly bodies (Figure 3.4) are remnant frag-

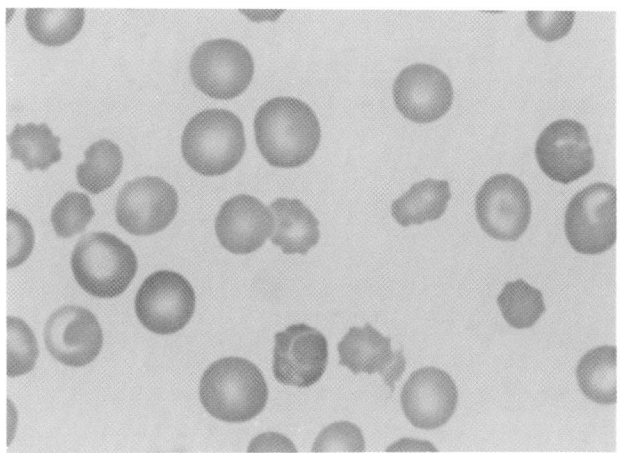

Figure 3.1. Polychromatophils. The bluish-staining, usually larger red blood cells are polychromatophils. In most animals, except horses, polychromatophils are present in high numbers in circulation during a regenerative anemia. In addition, there is slight poikilocytosis and target cells are present. Canine blood smear; 100× objective.

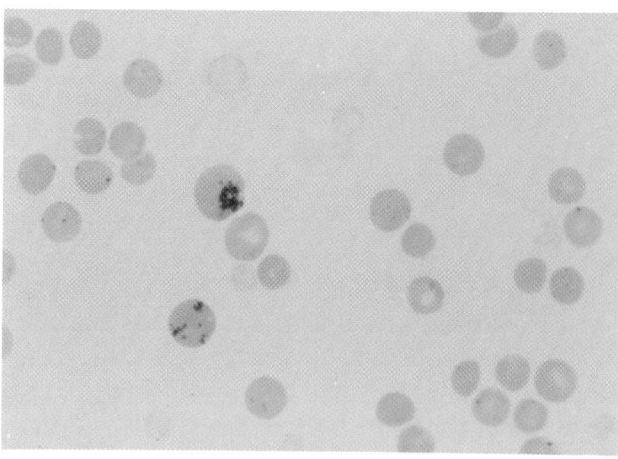

Figure 3.3. Aggregate and punctate reticulocytes. The two cells (left center) that have dark blue, clumped granular material in the cytoplasm are aggregate reticulocytes. The cells with small single or multiple dots of bluish material are punctate reticulocytes. The cells with no reticulum are mature red blood cells. Feline blood smear; new methylene blue stain; 100× objective.

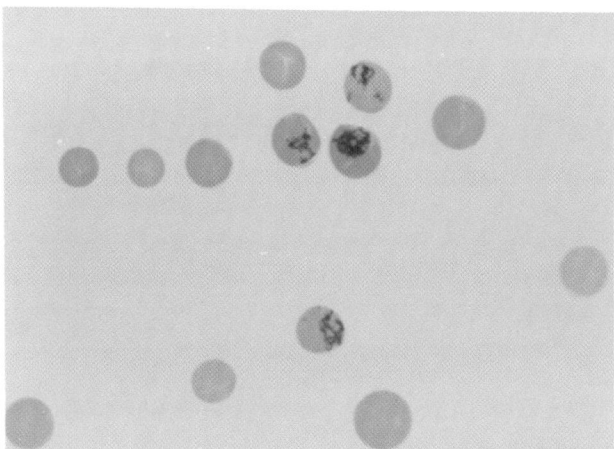

Figure 3.2. Reticulocytes. The four cells with dark blue, clumped granular material (reticulum) in the cytoplasm are reticulocytes. The cells with no reticulum are mature red blood cells. Canine blood smear; new methylene blue stain; 100× objective.

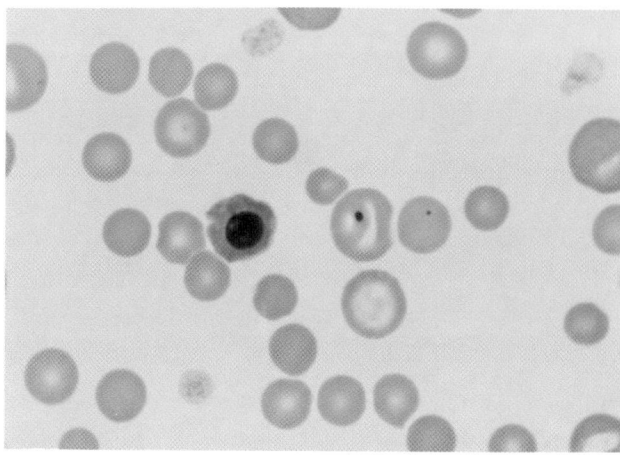

Figure 3.4. Nucleated red blood cell and Howell-Jolly bodies. The slightly blue cell with the round nucleus and condensed chromatin is a nucleated red blood cell (metarubricyte). Two adjacent red blood cells have single, small, round, deep purple cytoplasmic inclusions; these are Howell-Jolly bodies, which are fragments of nuclei. Canine blood smear; 100× objective.

ments of nuclear material present in red blood cells. Their presence during a regenerative response is probably due to the inability of macrophages to fully remove the nuclei of the maturing red blood cells during accelerated production. If Howell-Jolly bodies are present with a lack of adequate polychromasia, then decreased macrophagic function should be considered, especially splenic macrophagic function. A normal animal that has been splenectomized will often have Howell-Jolly bodies in circulation.

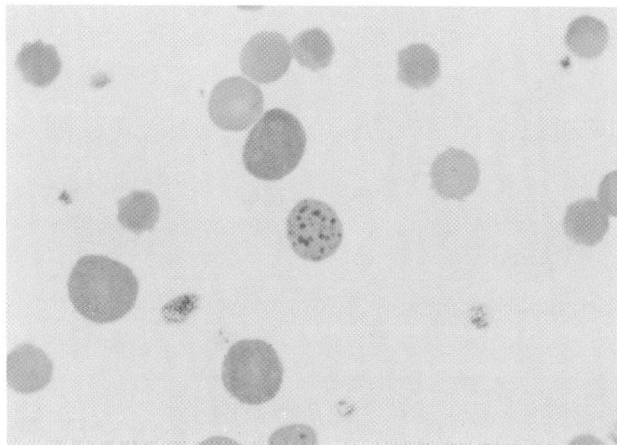

Figure 3.5. Basophilic stippling. The red blood cell (center) with multiple, small blue dots is a red blood cell with basophilic stippling. The three large, bluish-staining red blood cells are polychromatophils. There is moderate anisocytosis present also. Bovine blood smear; 100× objective.

IMMUNE-MEDIATED DAMAGE

Red blood cell morphological abnormalities associated with erythrocytic-directed immune-mediated processes result in the possibility of finding spherocytes, agglutination, and ghost cells. Spherocytes (Figure 3.6) are formed by macrophages partially removing antibody-coated membranes. Because of the membrane loss, these cells can no longer retain their normal discoid shape, thus a spherical shape with a lack of central pallor is produced. These cells are most easily recognized in dogs. Spherocytes are difficult to recognize in other species due to the lack of significant central pallor in their normal red blood cells. Sphero-

cytes may be present in low numbers when there is nonimmune-mediated damage to the red blood cells as well.

Agglutination (Figure 3.7) is an unorganized three-dimensional clustering of red blood cells, typically formed due to a cross-linking of red blood cell surface–associated antibodies. Agglutination also has been seen in horses that were treated with heparin. Agglutination may be seen both macroscopically and microscopically and must be distinguished from rouleaux formation (Figure 3.8), which is related to the charges on red blood cells.

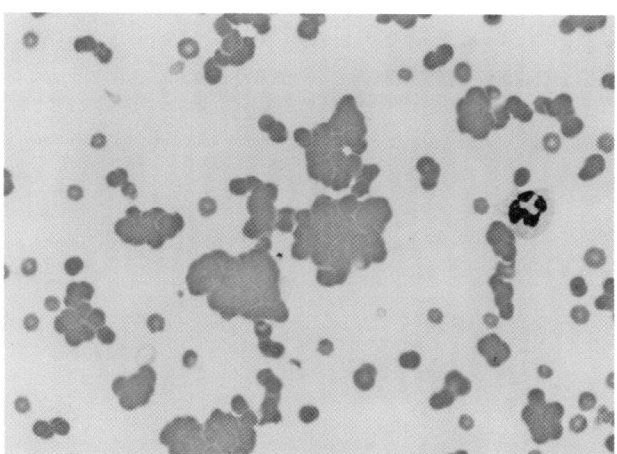

Figure 3.7. Agglutination. There are several irregular clusters of red blood cells present; this is agglutination. These are present throughout the field, but three large clumps are present (center). Agglutination may be seen in animals with immune-mediated anemia. Equine blood smear; 50× objective.

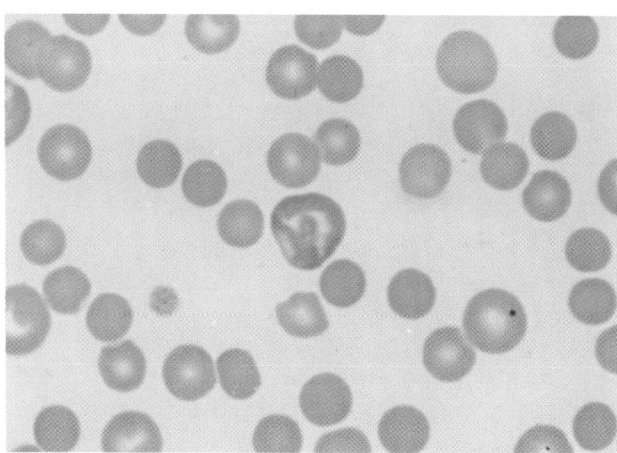

Figure 3.6. Spherocytes. The smaller cells that lack central pallor are spherocytes. These cells may be present in relatively high numbers in animals with immune-mediated hemolytic anemia. There is also a polychromatophil (center), and a red blood cell (lower right) with a Howell-Jolly body. Canine blood smear; 100× objective.

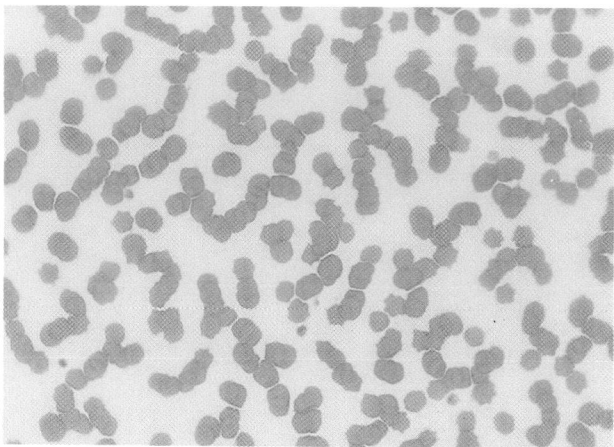

Figure 3.8. Rouleaux. The linear and sometimes branching chains of red blood cells is rouleaux formation. Under normal conditions, this finding is most prominent in horses; however, rouleaux may be seen in increased amounts associated with inflammatory disease in most species. Equine blood smear; 50× objective.

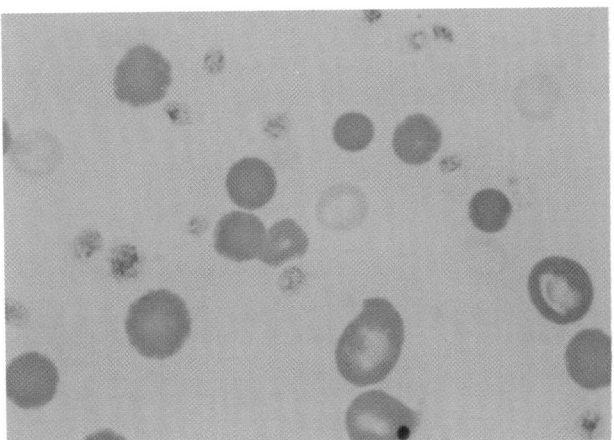

Figure 3.9. Ghost cells. The four very pale, small red blood cells are ghost cells. These indicate intravascular hemolysis. Also visible are spherocytes, polychromatophils, and a red blood cell with a large Howell-Jolly body. Canine blood smear; 100× objective.

Ghost cells (Figure 3.9) are remnant membranes of red blood cells that have undergone intravascular lysis. This lysis can be induced by binding antibody and complement to the red blood cell membrane as well as other nonimmune-mediated mechanisms.

OXIDATIVE INJURY

Oxidation of red blood cells may occur during some disease states, as well as with exposure to certain drugs. This oxidation and denaturation of hemoglobin in red blood cells results in the formation of protuberances from the red blood cell membrane that are often refractile; these are known as Heinz bodies (Figures 3.10 and 3.11). If the Heinz bodies are large, they

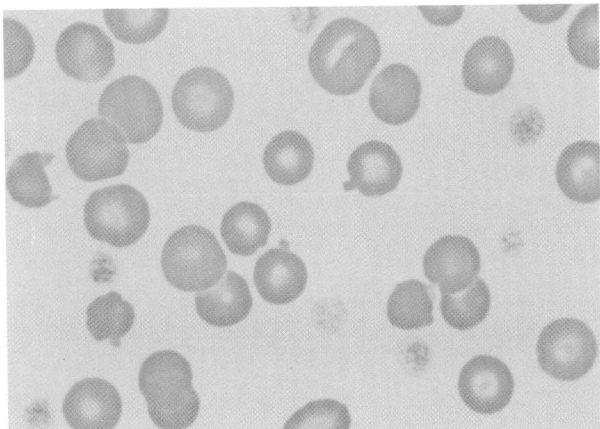

Figure 3.10. Heinz bodies. The small round projections from the surface of the red blood cells (center) are Heinz bodies. These represent oxidation and denaturation of hemoglobin. Canine blood smear; 100× objective.

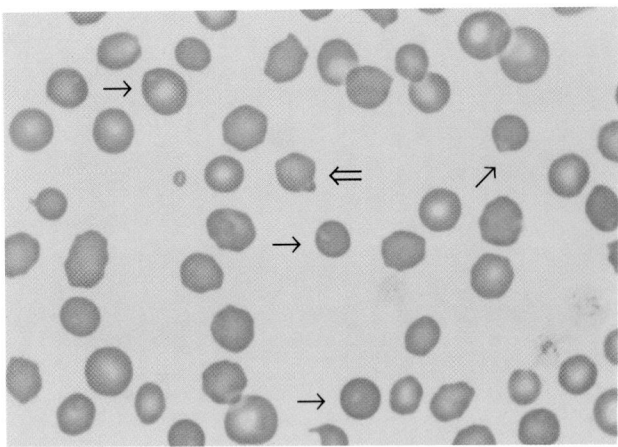

Figure 3.11. Heinz bodies. The red blood cell (double arrow) has a small round projection from the surface at the 5 o'clock position that is a Heinz body. Many of the red blood cells also have small, round clear structures on their surface (single arrows) that are also Heinz bodies. Feline blood smear; 100× objective.

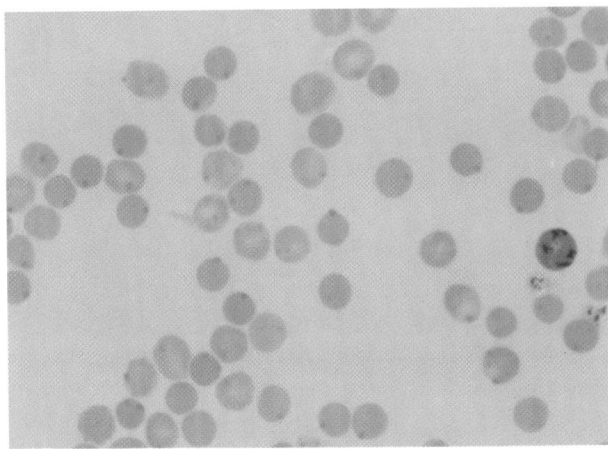

Figure 3.12. Heinz bodies. The red blood cell (center) has a Heinz body, which is the small, round, light blue-green projection from the surface at the 12 o'clock position. Many of the red blood cells throughout the field also have single, or sometimes multiple, Heinz bodies. There is also an aggregate reticulocyte (right center). Feline blood smear; new methylene blue stain; 100× objective.

can easily be seen on Wright's-stained smears. These structures can also be identified using new methylene blue–stained smears in which they stain light greenish-blue (Figure 3.12). Heinz bodies are often seen more commonly in cats.

Another cell type that is sometimes present upon exposure to oxidants is the eccentrocyte (Figure 3.13). These cells have crescent-shaped clear areas that are eccentrically placed. This clear area represents where cell membranes are closely apposed and possibly bonded due to oxidant-induced membrane damage.

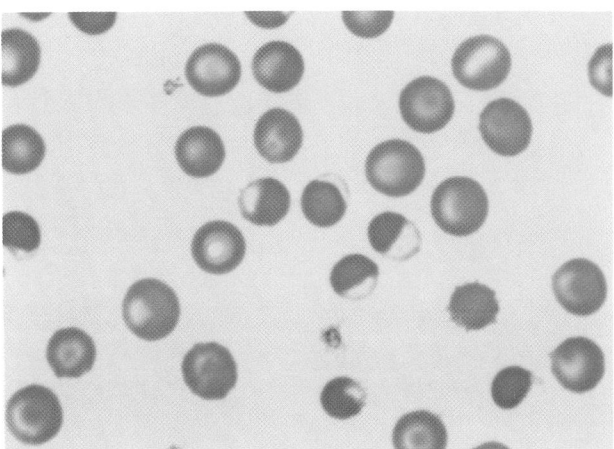

Figure 3.13. Eccentrocytes. The four red blood cells (center) with peripheral clear areas and displaced hemoglobin are eccentrocytes. Others are located at the periphery of the field. These represent oxidation of red blood cell membranes. Canine blood smear; 100× objective.

METABOLIC/MEMBRANE DISORDERS

Exposure of red blood cells to different environments, both in vitro and in vivo, can result in morphological variations from the normal discoid shape. One of the more common variations seen is the echinocyte. Echinocytes are cells with multiple, small, delicate, regular-shaped spines distributed evenly around red blood cell membranes. The most common cause for echinocyte formation is an in vitro artifact, crenation (Figure 3.14), which needs to be distinguished from true echinocytes. True echinocytes occur in association with different metabolic disorders such as renal disease. Collecting and immediately fixing blood prior to exposure to glass or an anticoagulant is required to distinguish true echinocytes from crenation.

Burr cells (Figure 3.15) have multiple projections similar to echinocytes but are oval to elongate. Burr cells may be seen in animals with renal disease.

In contrast to echinocytes, acanthocytes (Figure 3.16) are cells with multiple (2 to 10), irregularly shaped, blunt finger-like projections. These cells are formed due to alterations in the ratio of cholesterol

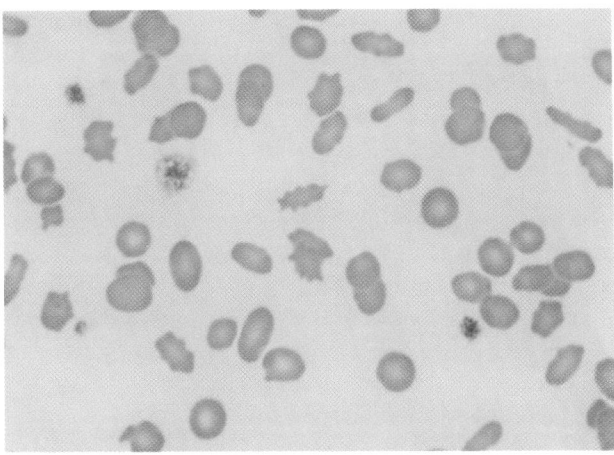

Figure 3.15. Burr cells. The elongated red blood cells with multiple, short blunt projections from the surface are burr cells. These cells may be seen in animals with renal disease. Feline blood smear; 100× objective.

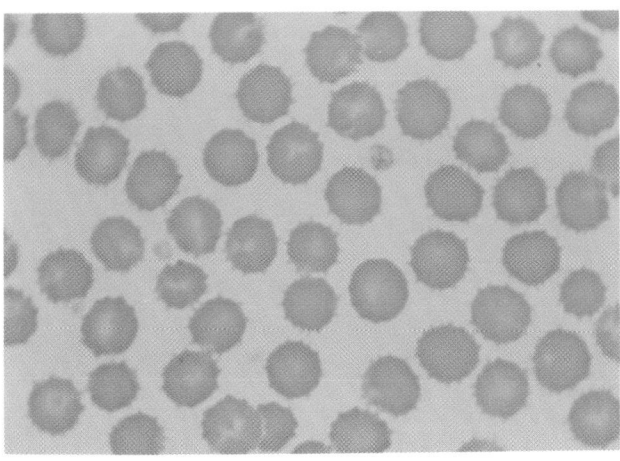

Figure 3.14. Echinocytes. The majority of the red blood cells have small uniform spines projecting from the surface. These are echinocytes. The most common cause of echinocyte formation is an in vitro artifact, known as crenation. Canine blood smear; 100× objective.

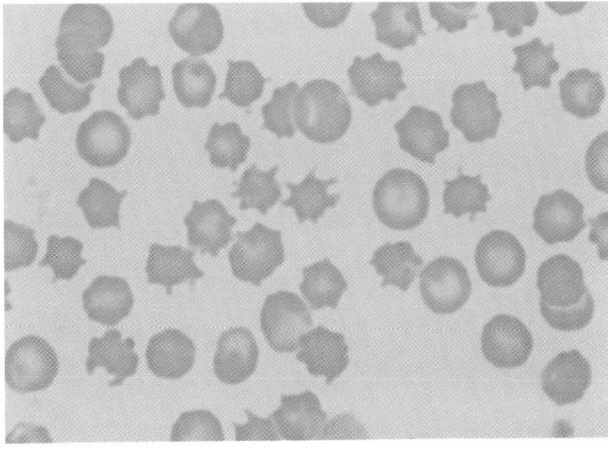

Figure 3.16. Acanthocytes. Note the red blood cells with multiple irregularly shaped projections from the surface. This abnormality is associated with alterations in cholesterol and phospholipid ratios in the membrane. These cells may be seen in animals with liver disease. Canine blood smear; 100× objective.

and phospholipid in the red blood cell membranes. Acanthocytes are commonly seen in animals with liver disease and are often seen in dogs with hemangiosarcoma; they may be due to neoplastic involvement of the liver or an unusual fragmentation due to the tortuosity of the neoplastic vasculature. Acanthocytes may also potentially be seen in association with renal disease–induced lipid abnormalities.

Keratocytes (Figure 3.17) are cells with two fairly uniform horn-like projections. These are thought to arise from a localized area of membrane damage in which a vacuole or "blister" is formed in the red blood cell membrane and which subsequently ruptures. The cells with intact blister-like membrane structures are commonly known as blister cells (Figure 3.18).

There are several potentially significant morphological changes associated with changes in the zone of central pallor. Two cell types that result in accentuation of the central pallor are hypochromic cells and torocytes. In hypochromic cells (Figures 3.19 and 3.20), there is increased central pallor, and the cells stain a lighter red due to a decreased amount of hemoglobin. As with normal red blood cells, there is a gradual transition between the outer and more dense staining regions of the cells and the central zone of pallor. Hypochromic cells are present in animals with iron deficiency, because iron is needed for normal hemoglobin synthesis. In contrast, in torocytes (Figure 3.21), although there is accentuated central pallor, the diameter of the central pallor region is not typically as great as that of hypochromic cells, the overall density of the red coloration of the cell is normal, and there is an abrupt transition between the outer and central

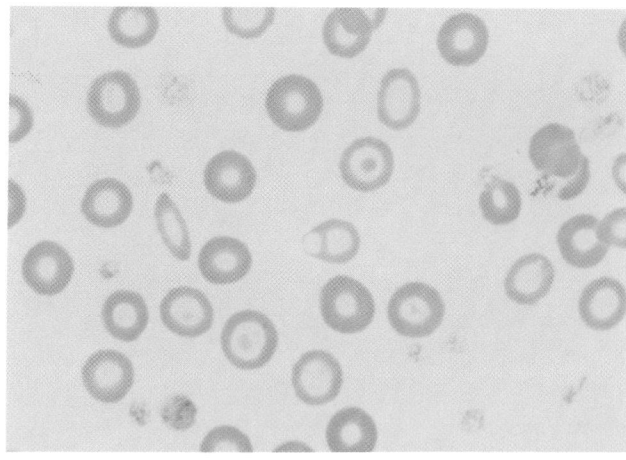

Figure 3.18. Blister cell. The cell with a thin piece of membrane extending from the surface (center) is a blister cell. This "blister" often ruptures to form a keratocyte. Hypochromic cells are also present. Canine blood smear; 100× objective.

zones of the cell. Torocytes are also commonly known as punched-out cells and are usually artifacts of preparation.

Stomatocytes (Figure 3.22) are cells in which the central pallor is more oval to elongate and takes on the appearance of a mouth. If these cells are evaluated in wet mount preparations, they are seen as being folded over on themselves in one direction. Stomatocytes have been seen in animals with red blood cell membrane metabolic defects, but they also can be found as an artifact of preparation in the thicker areas of the slide.

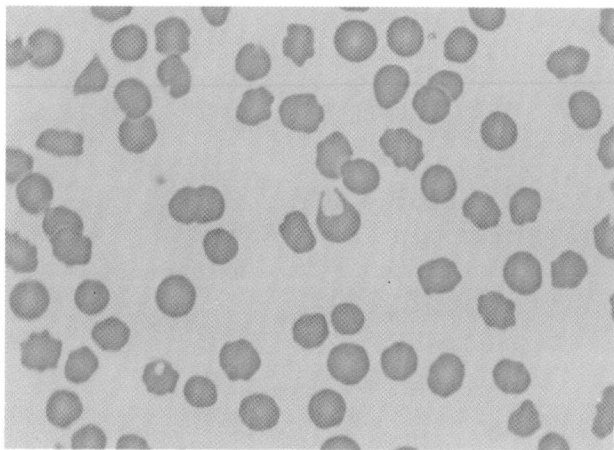

Figure 3.17. Keratocyte. The cell with two horn-like projections (center) is a keratocyte. Feline blood smear; 100× objective.

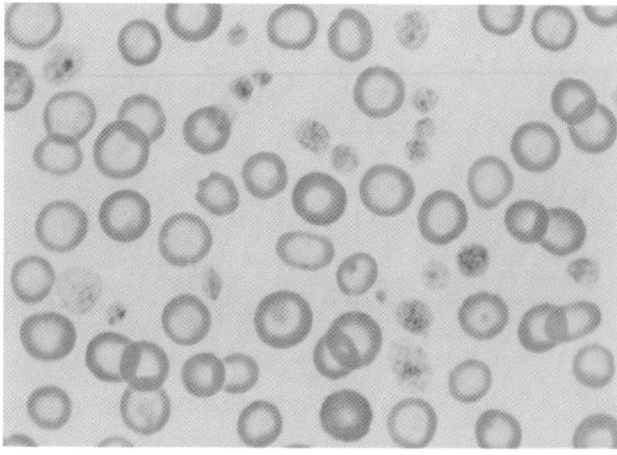

Figure 3.19. Hypochromic cells. There are several hypochromic cells throughout the field that have pronounced central pallor as well as faintly staining cell membranes. This change is most often associated with iron deficiency. Canine blood smear; 100× objective.

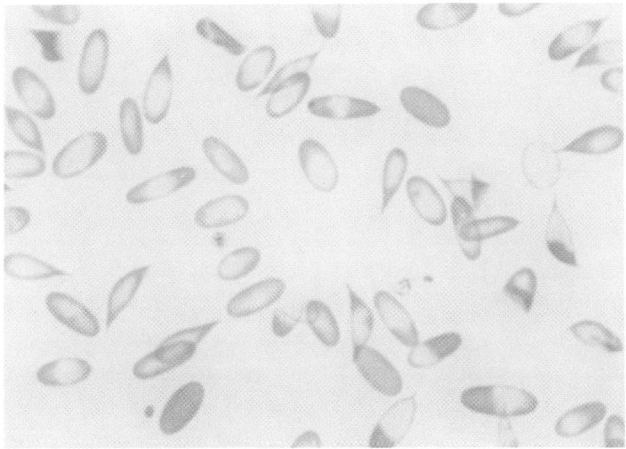

Figure 3.20. Hypochromic cells. The majority of the cells that have central pallor are hypochromic cells. A few normal llama red blood cells that typically lack central pallor are also present. This change is most often associated with iron deficiency. The fusiform shape of some of the cells is an additional common feature in llamas with iron deficiency. Llama blood smear; 100× objective.

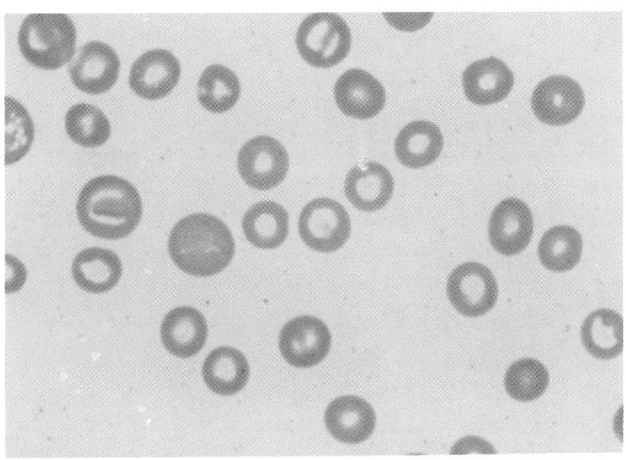

Figure 3.21. Torocyte. The majority of the cells in the field are torocytes, commonly known as punched-out cells. These cells have prominent central pallor with an abrupt transition from the pale center to the outer portion of the cell. They also may appear smaller than normal red blood cells. The torocyte morphology is typically an artifact resulting from abnormal spreading of cells on the slide. Canine blood smear; 100× objective.

Ovalocytes (Figure 3.23), also known as ellipto-cytes, are cells that are oval with an oval region of central pallor. They have been seen in animals with red blood cell membrane defects.

Leptocytes are cells that are larger than normal mature red blood cells and have excessively thin mem-

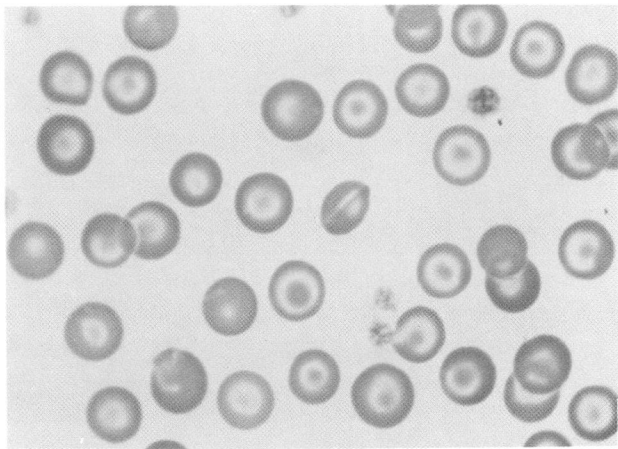

Figure 3.22. Stomatocyte. The somewhat oval cell with a linear central pallor (center) is a stomatocyte. Many target cells are also present. Canine blood smear; 100× objective.

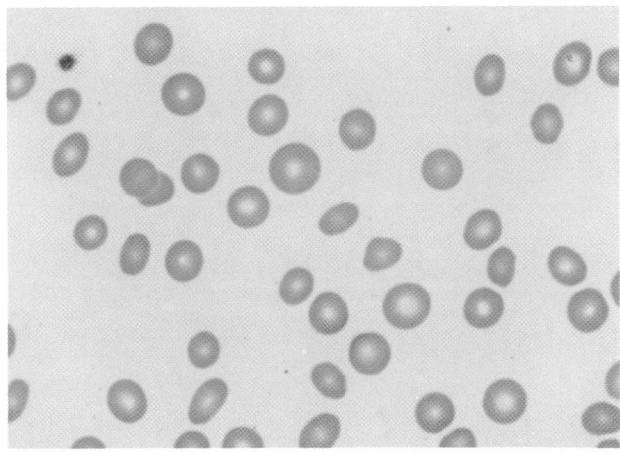

Figure 3.23. Ovalocytes. The oval red blood cells present are ovalocytes. They may be seen in animals with red blood cell membrane defects. Feline blood smear; 100× objective.

branes that tend to fold easily. Two types of leptocytes include target cells and bar cells.

Target cells (Figure 3.24), also known as codocytes, have an extra, round outfolding of the membrane in the middle of the cell that gives the cell a target-like appearance. Because polychromatophils often are very pliable, it is common for them to take on the appearance of a target cell. Target cell morphology is somewhat of a nonspecific change, but if it occurs in high numbers of mature red blood cells, investigation into possible liver disease should be considered.

Bar cells (Figure 3.25), also known as knizocytes, have a central bar-shaped outfolding of the membrane. Bar cells are often seen in similar situations as target cells.

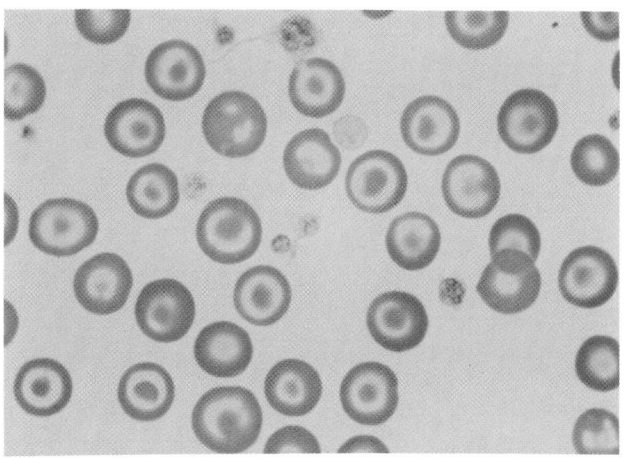

Figure 3.24. Target cells. Many of the red blood cells with a target-like appearance are target cells, also known as codocytes. The central area of the cells that stains represents an outfolding of the red blood cell membrane in this region. These cells may be found in animals with liver disease or with reticulocytosis. Canine blood smear; 100× objective.

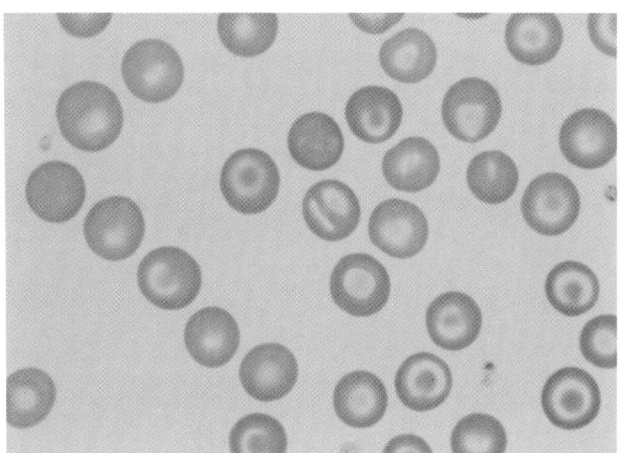

Figure 3.25. Bar cell. The cell (center) with a bar-shaped portion of membrane bisecting the area of central pallor is a bar cell, also known as a knizocyte. The change represents an outfolding of the red blood cell membrane similar to the change in the many target cells in this field. Canine blood smear; 100× objective.

MECHANICAL FRAGMENTATION

Schistocytes (Figure 3.26), also known as schizocytes, are fragments of red blood cells. These fragments result from mechanical damage to red blood cells in circulation, often due to microvascular abnormalities. One of the more common abnormalities that leads to schistocyte formation is the presence of fibrin

strands in the microvasculature. These strands can cut red blood cells into two or more irregularly shaped pieces as the cells traverse the vasculature. A common pathophysiological state in which these changes may be seen is disseminated intravascular coagulation.

Dacryocytes (Figure 3.27) are teardrop-shaped red blood cells. It is not exactly clear how these cells are formed, but this change may represent a type of fragmentation. They may be seen in animals with myelofibrosis.

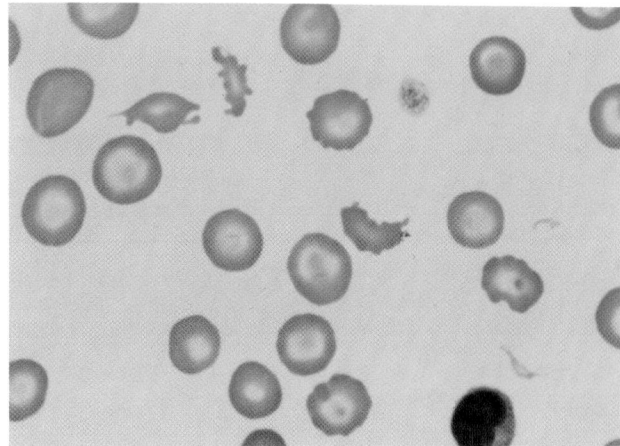

Figure 3.26. Schistocytes. The irregularly shaped red blood cell (center) is a schistocyte, or red blood cell fragment. There are two very small schistocytes in the lower right quadrant. Two much larger fragments are present (upper left). This change is related to mechanical damage to the red blood cell. Canine blood smear; 100× objective.

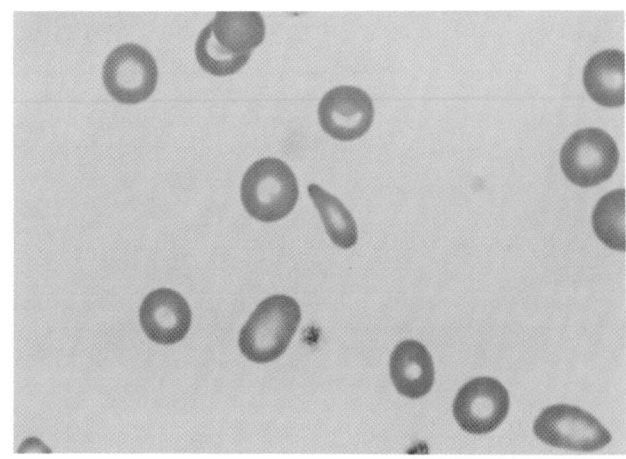

Figure 3.27. Dacryocyte. The teardrop-shaped red blood cell (center) is a dacryocyte. These cells may be seen in animals with myelofibrosis. Canine blood smear; 100× objective.

CHAPTER FOUR
RED BLOOD CELL
INCLUSIONS AND PARASITES

In evaluating red blood cells for inclusions or parasites, there are several normal structures and artifacts that often confuse the novice hematologist. Some of these structures were defined in Chapter 3 but are reviewed here briefly. One of the most common artifacts that is confused with red blood cell parasites or inclusions is stain precipitate (Figure 4.1), which presents as small, variably sized, pink to purple granular material. It often can be found on red blood cells as well as in the background of the slide; it is generally in a different plane of focus than the red blood cells. This distribution and size variability is helpful in distinguishing stain precipitate from true red blood cell parasites. In contrast, basophilic stippling (retained RNA aggregates) (Figure 4.2) appears as very small, multiple, round blue granules in the cytoplasm of the red blood cell. As previously stated in Chapter 3, this material is generally retained aggregates of RNA in the cell. Basophilic stippling is difficult to distinguish from Pappenheimer bodies, which are small blue granules in red blood cells. Pappenheimer bodies are aggregates of iron accumulation in the red blood cells (Figure 4.3). Anucleated and nucleated red blood cells with Pappenheimer bodies are known as siderocytes and sideroblasts respectively. A special stain, such as a Prussian blue, is the only way to confirm the presence of Pappenheimer bodies. When small blue granules

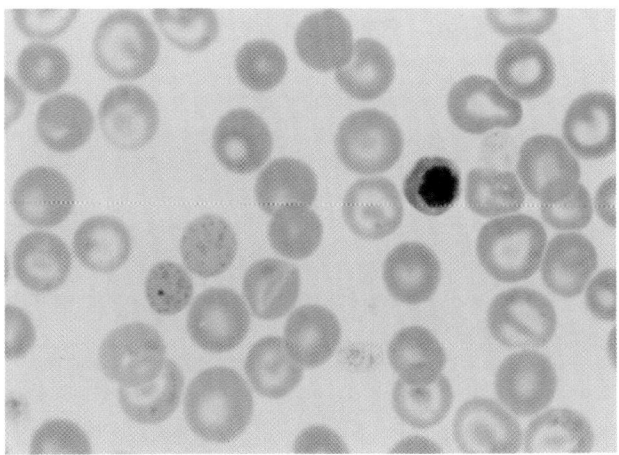

Figure 4.2. Basophilic stippling. Several of the red blood cells have very small, variably sized, pale blue granules, which are known as basophilic stippling. This is best demonstrated in the two red blood cells in the lower left quadrant. A metarubricyte is present in the upper right quadrant. Canine blood smear; 100× objective.

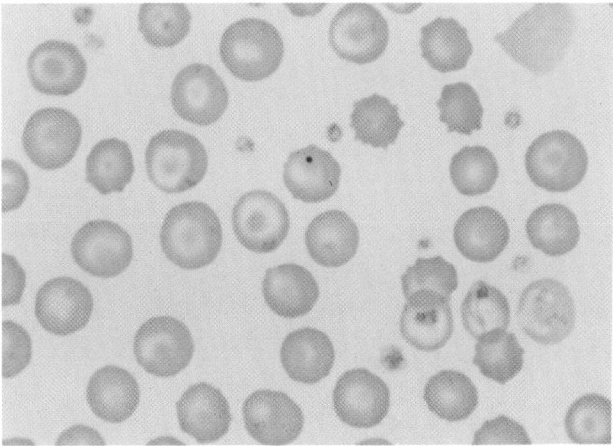

Figure 4.3. Pappenheimer bodies. The very small, poorly distinct, pale blue granules in some of the red blood cells are Pappenheimer bodies. These are best demonstrated in the three red blood cells that are in a row in the lower right quadrant. These inclusions are due to iron accumulation. In contrast, the red blood cell in the center of the field contains a small, round, deep purple structure, which is a Howell-Jolly body. Canine blood smear, from 1988 ASVCP slide review, courtesy of J. A. Matthews; 100× objective.

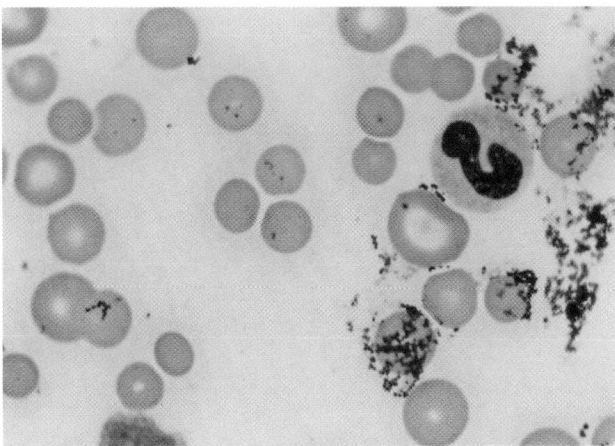

Figure 4.1. Stain precipitate. The variably sized, purple granular material present on and between the red blood cells is stain precipitate. Canine blood smear; 100× objective.

are present in the red blood cells, they are most likely basophilic stippling, not Pappenheimer bodies.

Another artifact that may be confused with erythrocytic parasites is red blood cell refractile artifacts. It is not clear how these form. This material can take on several sizes and shapes but can be confused with erythrocytic parasites when it is of similar size to such organisms as *Haemobartonella*. The main feature used to distinguish this artifact from a true parasite is that these structures are variably sized and refractile when the microscope is focused up and down (Figure 4.4).

Finally, occasionally platelets may be seen on top of red blood cells and thus appear to be inclusions (Figure 4.5). By comparing the platelet on top of the red blood cell with those platelets present throughout the rest of the slide, these should be distinguishable from true red cell inclusions or parasites.

Howell-Jolly bodies (Figure 4.6) are remnant micronuclei that may be seen in most domestic species during a regenerative anemia. These structures stain dark purple and are approximately 1 μm in diameter, although they can be larger. A single micronucleus typically is present in a red blood cell. In ruminants, *Anaplasma* organisms (Figure 4.7) can look very similar in size, shape, and staining intensity to Howell-Jolly bodies. Fortunately, the most common type of anaplasmosis is due to *Anaplasma marginale*, which as the name implies, is often found at the periphery of the red blood cell. Although Howell-Jolly bodies can be found on the edge of the cell, the majority of these structures are more randomly distributed in the red blood cells. In addition, in anaplasmosis, more than one organism per cell is often present, whereas with Howell-Jolly bodies, the micronuclei are usually singular. Because anaplasmosis often causes a regenerative anemia, both *Anaplasma* and Howell-Jolly bodies may be present concurrently.

Viral inclusions can be found in red blood cells (Figure 4.8) and white blood cells in dogs with distemper virus infection. These inclusions are quite variable in size, but usually are much larger than Howell-Jolly bodies. Viral inclusions can be several microns in diameter and are round to oblong to quite variably shaped. They typically stain pink to red, although more-bluish inclusions have been reported. There is

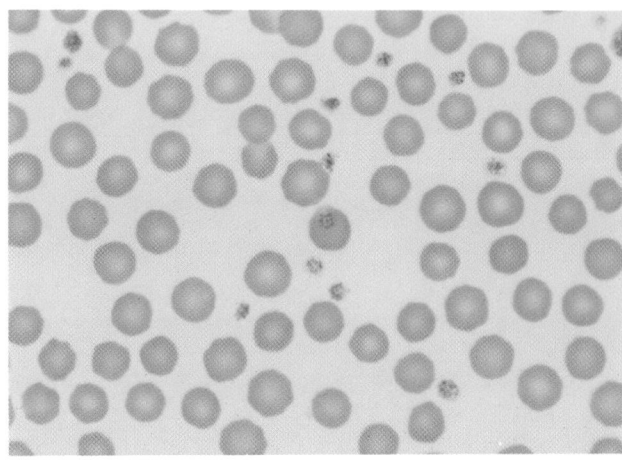

Figure 4.5. Erythrocyte pseudoinclusion. A platelet superimposed on a red blood cell is present in the center of the field. Note the similar features to the other platelets. Bovine blood smear; 100× objective.

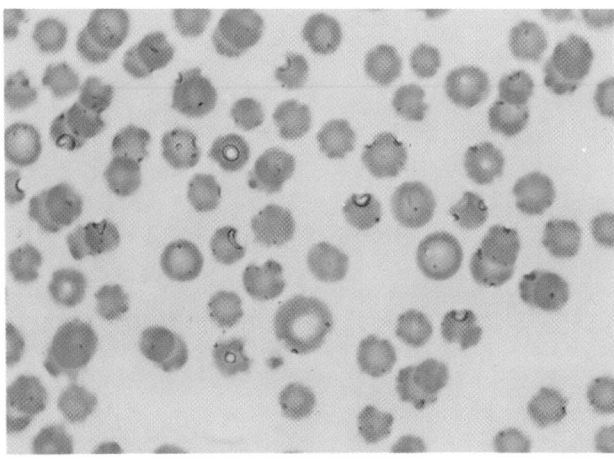

Figure 4.4. Refractile artifact. The round to oval, or irregularly shaped and variably sized, shiny unstained structures present on the surface of the red blood cells are refractile artifacts. Bovine blood smear; 100× objective.

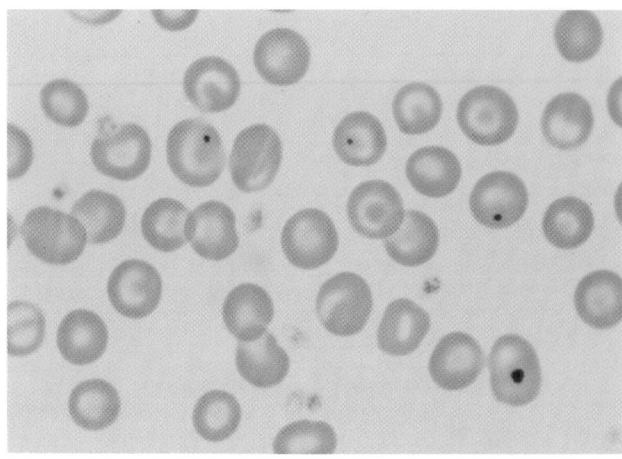

Figure 4.6. Howell-Jolly bodies. Four red blood cells have single, small, round, deep purple cytoplasmic inclusions; these are Howell-Jolly bodies, which are nuclear fragments. Target cells are also present. Canine blood smear; 100× objective.

no real internal structure, and often the inclusion has a smooth glassy appearance, but it may be granular. Diff-Quik® stain is often stated as the preferred stain for identifying viral inclusions.

The common red blood cell parasites of dogs are *Haemobartonella canis* and *Babesia canis*. *H. canis* (Figure 4.9) is a very small epicellular parasite, less than 1 μm in diameter, and may be difficult to distinguish from stain artifact. It is coccoid or rod shaped and can be found individually or in groups on red blood cells. The organism often forms chains across the red blood cells. Babesiosis is most commonly caused by *Babesia canis* (Figure 4.10) and is found mainly in the south-

eastern United States, South and Central America, Southern Europe, Africa, Asia, and Australia. This large, intracellular, pyriform-shaped parasite is easy to recognize, although often very few cells in a blood smear contain organisms. These organisms are typically 2.5 to 3 μm wide by 4 to 5 μm long. Multiple organisms may be present in the cell. *B. gibsoni* (U.S.A., Southern Europe, Asia) also causes disease in dogs and is typically a much smaller, round to oval to elongate organism.

The most common red blood cell parasite of cats is *Haemobartonella felis* (Figure 4.11). This small coccoid- to rod-shaped epicellular organism is similar in mor-

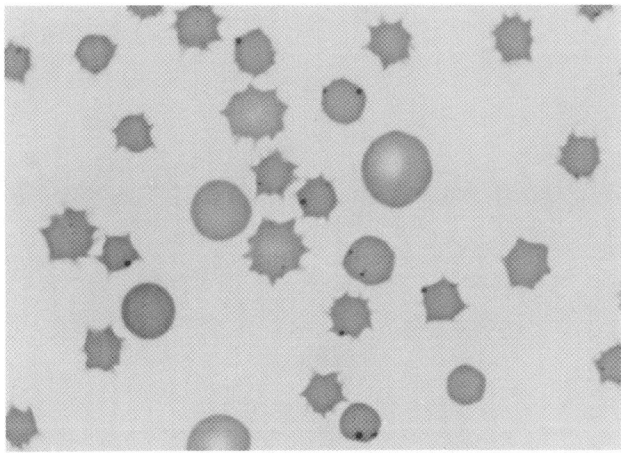

Figure 4.7. *Anaplasma marginale.* The single to multiple, round, deep purple cytoplasmic inclusions in several of the red blood cells are *Anaplasma marginale* organisms. Note that many of these organisms are present on the extreme periphery of the red blood cell. Bovine blood smear; 100× objective.

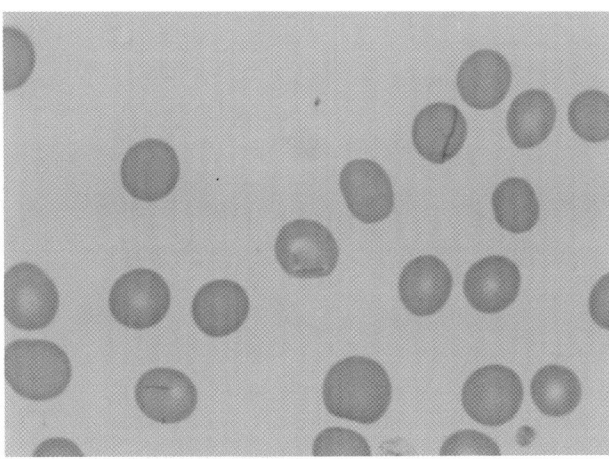

Figure 4.9. *Haemobartonella canis.* The very small, coccoid- to rod-shaped blue structures forming chains on several of the red blood cells are *Haemobartonella canis* organisms. Canine blood smear; 100× objective.

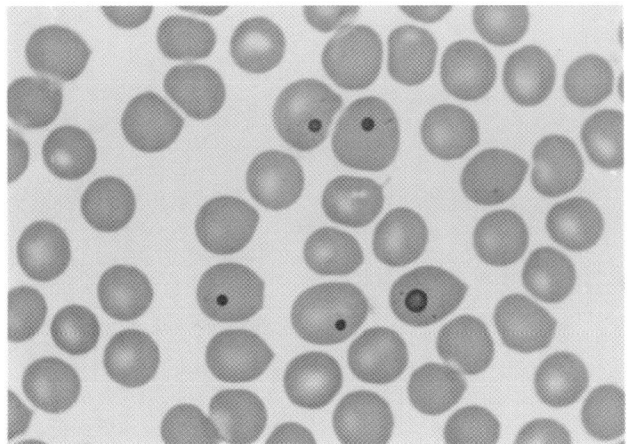

Figure 4.8. Distemper viral inclusions. The variably sized, round, reddish-pink structures present in five of the red blood cells are canine distemper viral inclusions. Canine blood smear; 100× objective.

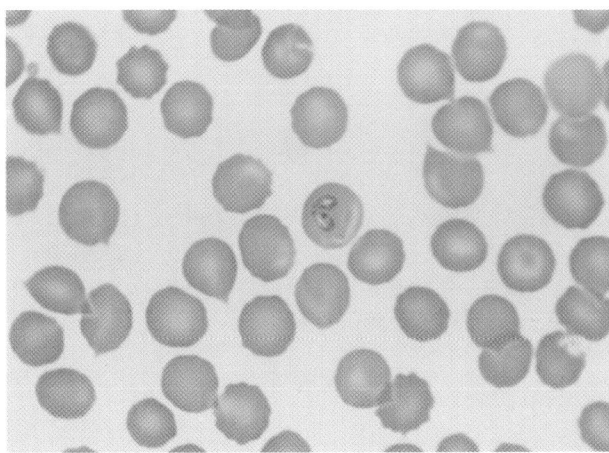

Figure 4.10. *Babesia canis.* There are two *Babesia canis* organisms within the red blood cell in the middle of the field. These are light blue pyriform structures with poorly defined internal purple bodies. Canine blood smear; Diff-Quik® stain; 100× objective.

phology to *H. canis*. In addition, ring forms also may be seen. As with *H. canis*, *H. felis* can be difficult to distinguish from stain precipitate. It requires a good-quality, well-stained blood smear for accurate identification. Attachment of the organisms to the outside of the cell is not very strong, thus the organisms can be removed easily. If there is a delay in making an air-dried blood smear from EDTA anticoagulated blood, organisms may be found in the background of the slide and not on the red blood cells.

Cytauxzoon felis (Figure 4.12) is another red blood cell parasite of cats. It is often bluish-staining and oval (1 to 5 μm in diameter) with a clear central region. Often a purple nucleus is on one end of the oval, giving the organism a signet ring appearance. Some organisms have chromatin bodies on both ends, giving them a "safety pin" appearance. Typically, these organisms are present in the blood in low numbers. Most cases have been reported in Missouri, the southern United States, and South and Central America.

In ruminants, *Anaplasma* (U.S.A. and tropical areas) and *Babesia* (Northern and Western Europe) are the most common red blood cell parasites. In cattle, anaplasmosis is most often caused by *Anaplasma marginale* (Figure 4.7). These organisms are approximately 1 μm in diameter, are coccoid shaped, stain dark purple, and are often located on the periphery of the red blood cells; one to a few organisms may be present per red blood cell. As stated earlier, these organisms must be distinguished from Howell-Jolly bodies. In an infected animal, many red blood cells usually contain the parasite.

Another parasite of ruminants, as well as of llamas, is *Eperythrozoon* (Figure 4.13). *E. wenyoni* (U.S.A. and Africa) is the organism that typically infects cattle; *E. ovis* affects sheep worldwide. In llamas the exact species of the organism has not been determined. In both ruminants and llamas, the organisms look very similar to *Haemobartonella felis*. These organisms can appear as coccoid- or rod-shaped or ring-like structures on the surface of the red blood cell. They are approximately 0.5 μm in diameter. Multiple organisms are often found on red blood cells, and organisms may be found in the background of the slide as well.

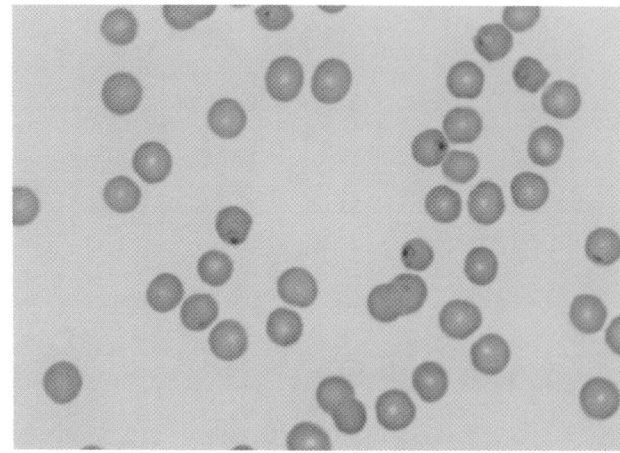

Figure 4.12. *Cytauxzoon felis.* Three red blood cells in the center of the field have blue rings, each with a single, eccentrically located purple nucleus. These organisms are *Cytauxzoon felis.* A few additional red blood cells with less-distinct organisms are also present. Feline blood smear, courtesy of G. D. Boon; 100× objective.

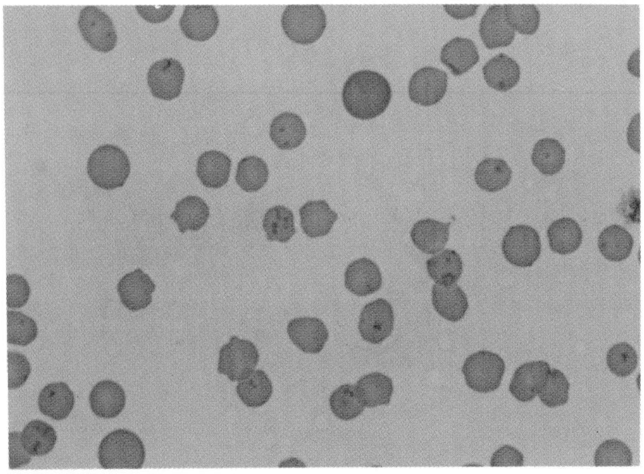

Figure 4.11. *Haemobartonella felis.* Many of the red blood cells have single or multiple; small; blue coccoid-, rod-, or ring-shaped organisms on their surface. These organisms are *Haemobartonella felis.* Feline blood smear; 100× objective.

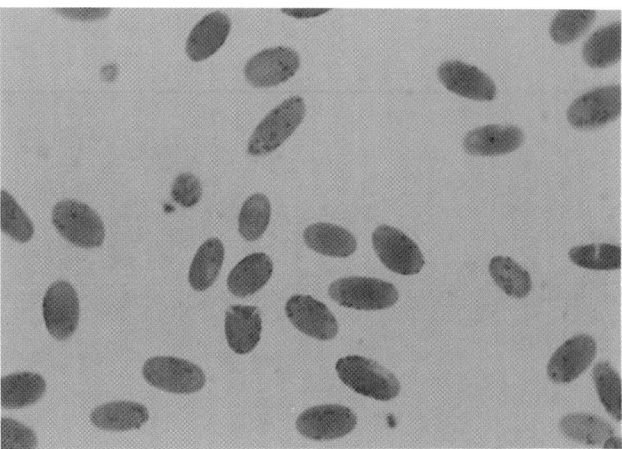

Figure 4.13. *Eperythrozoon.* The single or multiple; small; blue coccoid-, rod-, or ring-shaped organisms on the surface of these red blood cells are *Eperythrozoon.* Llama blood smear; 100× objective.

CHAPTER FIVE

NORMAL WHITE BLOOD CELL MORPHOLOGY

SEGMENTED NEUTROPHIL

Segmented neutrophils are the most common white blood cells in peripheral blood of all the common domestic species, except ruminants. Segmented neutrophils are typically 10 to 12 μm in diameter and have single nuclei with several indentations resulting in the nucleus being divided into multiple lobes. Typically there are 3 to 5 lobes or segments per cell. The chromatin pattern of the nucleus consists of very dark, condensed areas intermixed with small clear areas. The cytoplasm stains faintly blue to pink depending on the type and quality of the stain used. Sometimes very indistinct pink granules may be seen in the cytoplasm. The neutrophils of the different species look very similar. The major exception is that the cytoplasm of bovine neutrophils often stains more pink compared with that of the other species. Also, in horses, the segments of the nucleus are generally not as distinct.

BAND NEUTROPHIL

Band neutrophils may be absent or present in the peripheral blood in very low numbers. Band neutrophils look similar to segmented neutrophils except that the nuclei are band shaped. Classically, the nuclear membranes are parallel so that the nucleus has a constant width. Because band neutrophils are a stage in the gradual differentiation toward the segmented-neutrophil form, slight nuclear indentations are possible.

LYMPHOCYTE

Lymphocytes are the second most common cell type in the peripheral blood of most of the domestic species and are the most common cell type in ruminants. Typically, these cells are round, slightly smaller than neutrophils, and have round to oval and sometimes slightly indented nuclei. The chromatin pattern consists of smooth glassy areas intermixed with areas that are more clumped or smudged. A small amount of light blue cytoplasm is present. A few of the lymphocytes may have multiple, small, pinkish-purple granules in the cytoplasm. In addition to these small lymphocytes, many animals may have some medium to large lymphocytes. This is especially true for ruminants. Often these cells have more cytoplasm than small lymphocytes. In addition, the chromatin of ruminant nuclei is often much more accentuated with sometimes marked areas of condensation. This may lead to the false conclusion that nucleoli are present in these cells.

MONOCYTE

Monocytes are absent or present in low numbers in the peripheral blood and look very similar in all the common domestic species. These cells are typically 15 to 20 μm in diameter, and the nuclei can be different shapes: oval, oval with a single indentation (kidney bean–shaped), or have multiple indentations and lobulations. The nuclear chromatin is finely granular to lacy in appearance with only a few areas of condensation. The moderate amount of cytoplasm is typically blue-gray and may have multiple, variably sized discrete vacuoles.

EOSINOPHIL

Eosinophils are absent or present in very low numbers in normal animals. These cells are typically similar in size to neutrophils or slightly larger. The nuclei are very similar to those of neutrophils in that they are segmented, but the segments are often not as well defined. The cytoplasm stains faint blue and has multiple reddish to reddish-orange granules. The number and shapes of the granules are quite different for most of the common domestic species. Dog eosinophilic granules are round and quite variable in size and number. There are often multiple, variably sized vacuoles in the cytoplasm as well. Cat eosinophilic granules are rod shaped and typically fill the cytoplasm. Horse eosinophils have very large round, oval, or oblong granules that fill the cytoplasm and often obscure the nucleus. Ruminant eosinophils have small round, fairly uniform granules that typically fill the cytoplasm. Llama eosinophils have small round, oval, or oblong granules. The low number of granules typically does not fill the cytoplasm.

BASOPHIL

Basophils are rarely seen in the peripheral blood of all the common domestic species. They are most commonly seen in horses. Basophils are similar in size or slightly larger than neutrophils, and the cytoplasm is light purple. The nucleus is segmented but often not to the degree of the mature neutrophil. Low numbers of small, round, purple cytoplasmic granules may sometimes be present in dog basophils. The presence or absence of granules may be dependent on the type of stain used. Cat basophils contain indistinct small, round, lavender granules. Both cow and horse basophils have several small, well-stained purple granules in the cytoplasm. Llama basophils look very similar to cow or horse basophils. Figures 5.1–5.30 show the normal white blood cells of the common domestic species.

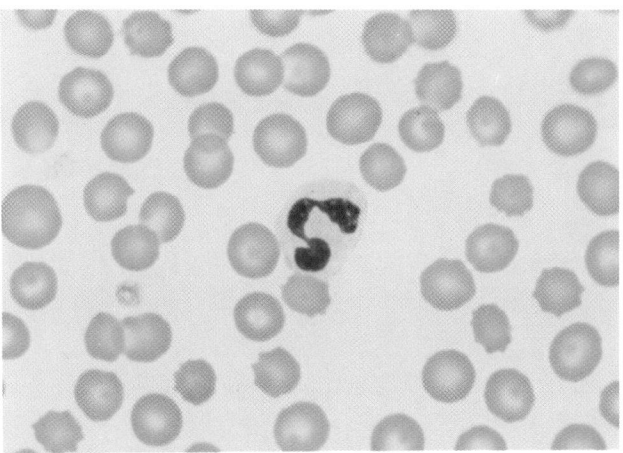

Figure 5.1. Segmented neutrophil. The cell with the segmented nucleus and pink cytoplasm is a mature neutrophil. Canine blood smear; 100× objective.

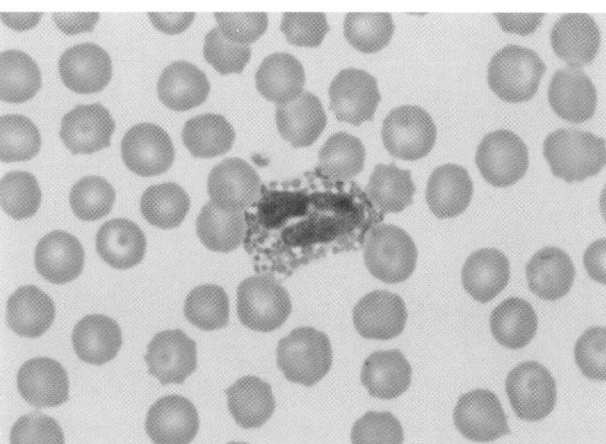

Figure 5.4. Eosinophil. The cell with a poorly segmented nucleus and multiple, round reddish granules in the cytoplasm is an eosinophil. Canine blood smear; 100× objective.

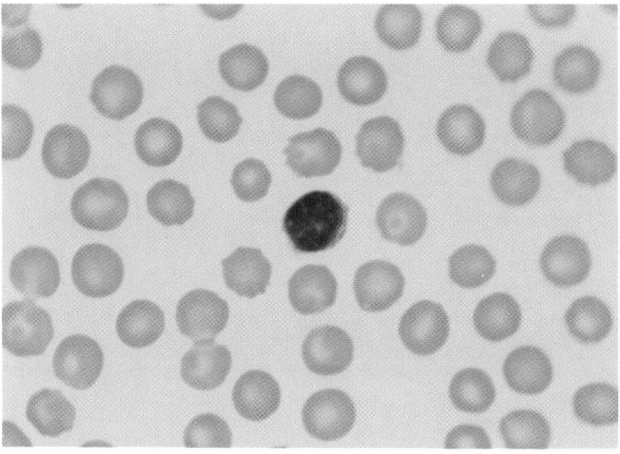

Figure 5.2. Small lymphocyte. The small cell with a round, centrally located nucleus and rim of light blue cytoplasm is a small lymphocyte. Canine blood smear; 100× objective.

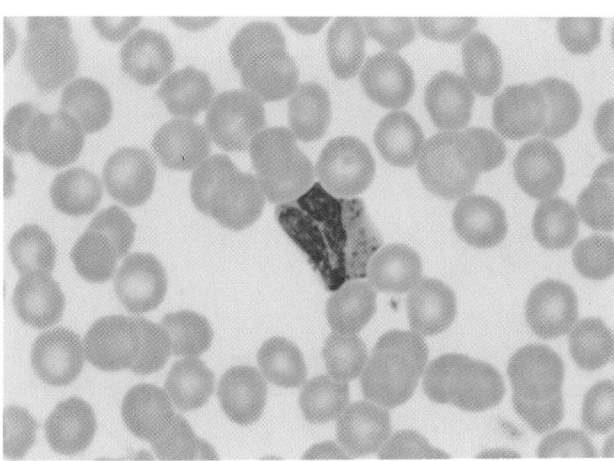

Figure 5.5. Basophil. The cell with the poorly segmented nucleus and light purple cytoplasm with low numbers of small, discrete purple granules is a basophil. Canine blood smear; 100× objective.

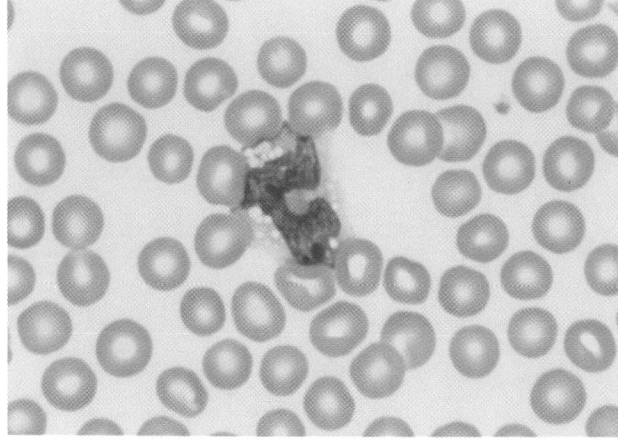

Figure 5.3. Monocyte. The large cell with a deeply indented nucleus, blue-gray cytoplasm, and multiple, discrete cytoplasmic vacuoles is a monocyte. Note the nucleus is not as prominently segmented as the mature neutrophil. Canine blood smear; 100× objective.

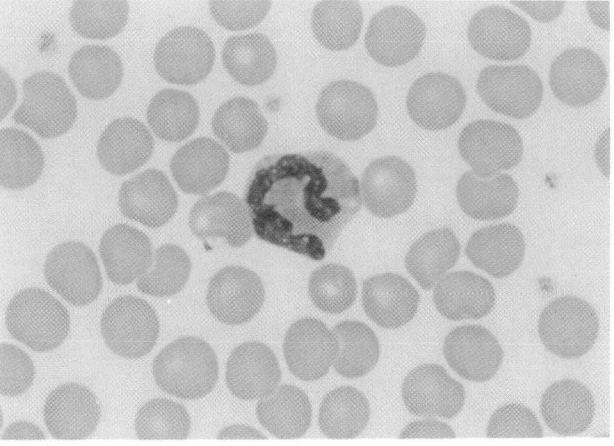

Figure 5.6. Basophil. The cell with the poorly segmented nucleus and light purple cytoplasm is a basophil. Without distinct granules, these cells can be difficult to distinguish from toxic neutrophils or monocytes. Canine blood smear; 100× objective.

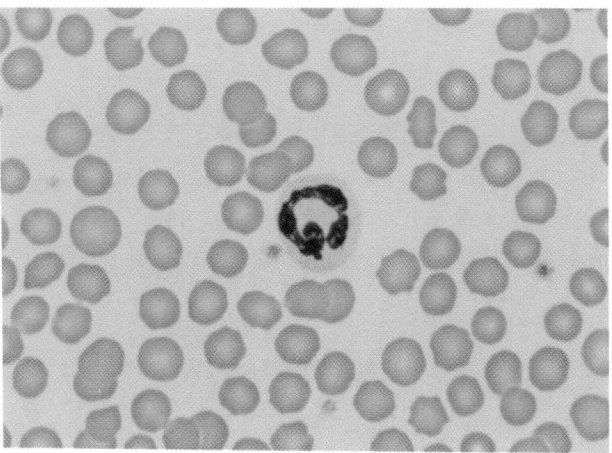

Figure 5.7. Segmented neutrophil. The cell with a segmented nucleus and light pink cytoplasm is a mature neutrophil. Feline blood smear; 100× objective.

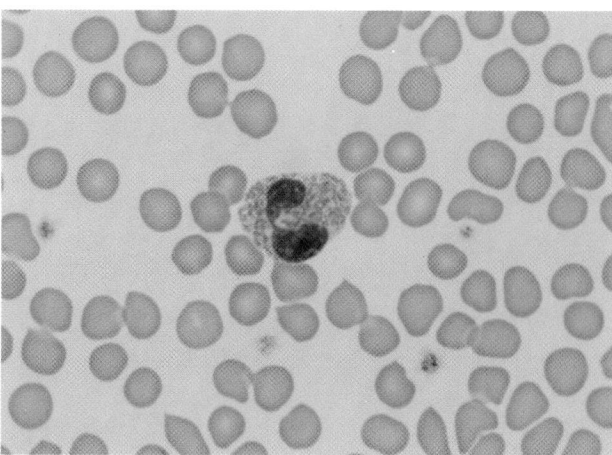

Figure 5.10. Eosinophil. The cell with a segmented nucleus and multiple, reddish rod-shaped granules in the cytoplasm is an eosinophil. Feline blood smear; 100× objective.

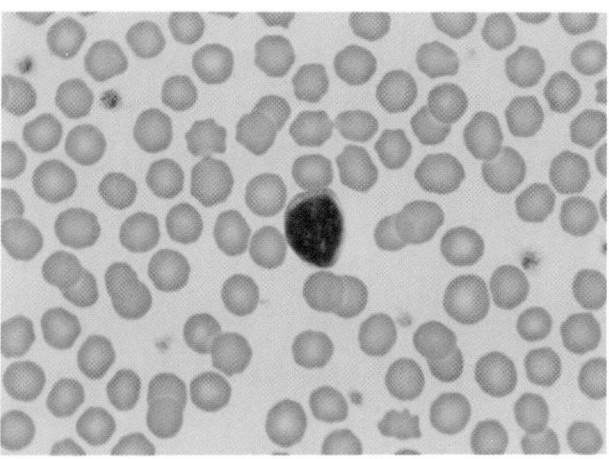

Figure 5.8. Small lymphocyte. The small cell with a round to oval, centrally located nucleus and rim of light blue cytoplasm is a small lymphocyte. Feline blood smear; 100× objective.

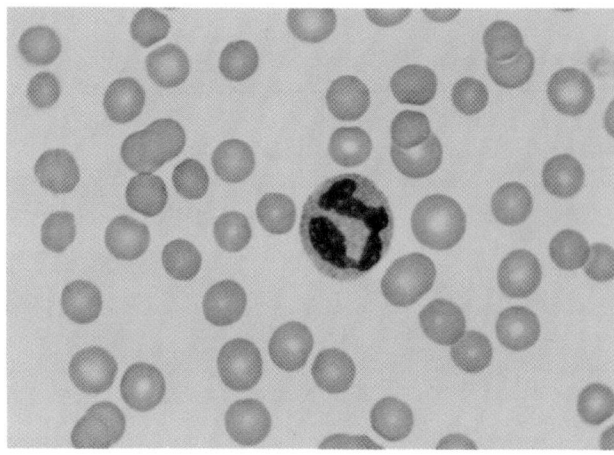

Figure 5.11. Basophil. The cell with a segmented nucleus and poorly defined, round, light purple granules in the cytoplasm is a basophil. Feline blood smear; 100× objective.

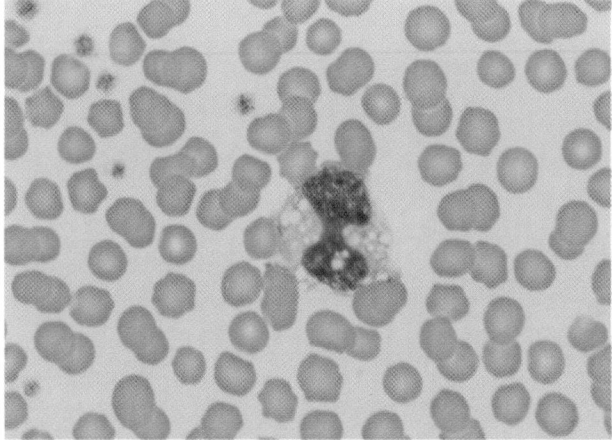

Figure 5.9. Monocyte. The large cell with a deeply indented nucleus, blue-gray cytoplasm, and multiple, discrete cytoplasmic vacuoles is a monocyte. Feline blood smear; 100× objective.

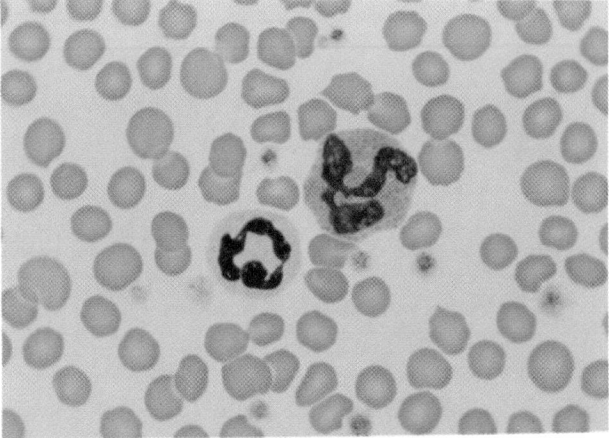

Figure 5.12. Segmented neutrophil and basophil. The cell to the lower left is a segmented neutrophil, and the cell to the upper right is a basophil. Note the slightly larger size of the basophil as well as the poorly defined, round, light purple cytoplasmic granules. Feline blood smear; 100× objective.

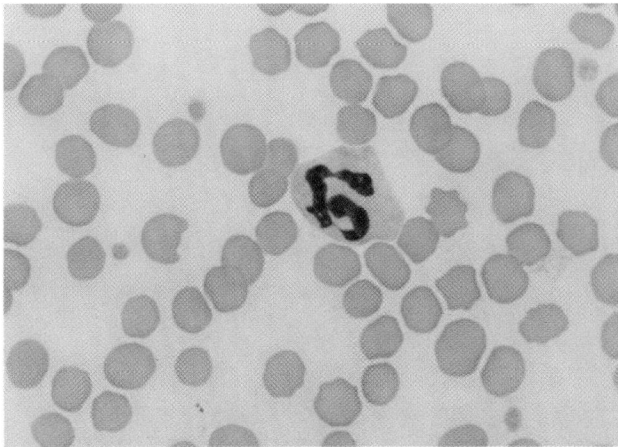

Figure 5.13. Segmented neutrophil. The cell with a segmented nucleus and light blue to pink cytoplasm is a mature neutrophil. Equine blood smear; 100× objective.

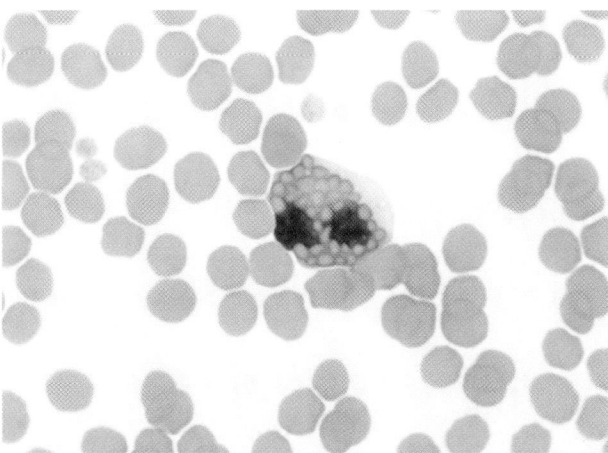

Figure 5.16. Eosinophil. The cell with the bilobed nucleus and very large, round to oval reddish granules in the cytoplasm is an eosinophil. Note that the granules are obscuring part of the nucleus. Equine blood smear; 100× objective.

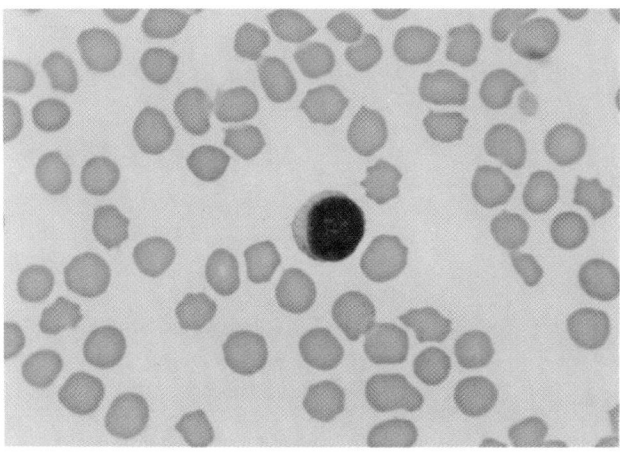

Figure 5.14. Small lymphocyte. The small cell with a round nucleus and a rim of light blue cytoplasm is a small lymphocyte. Equine blood smear; 100× objective.

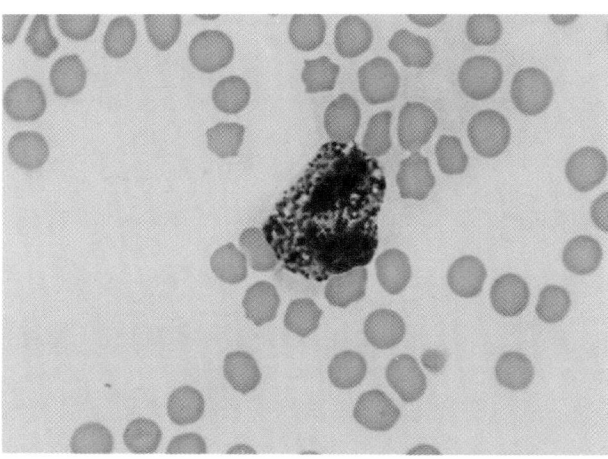

Figure 5.17. Basophil. The cell with bilobed nucleus and numerous small, purple cytoplasmic granules is a basophil. Note that the granules are obscuring part of the nucleus. Equine blood smear; 100× objective.

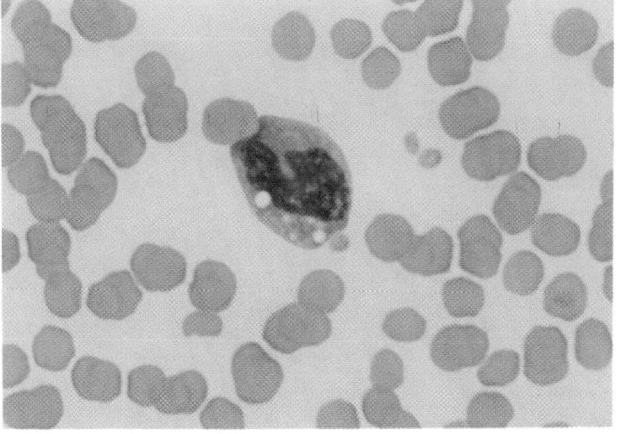

Figure 5.15. Monocyte. The large cell with a deeply indented nucleus, blue-gray cytoplasm, and multiple, discrete cytoplasmic vacuoles is a monocyte. Equine blood smear; 100× objective.

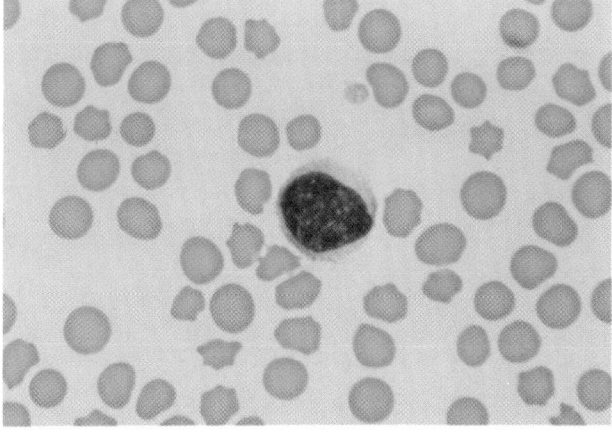

Figure 5.18. Large lymphocyte. The large round cell with an oval nucleus and a rim of light blue cytoplasm is a large lymphocyte. Equine blood smear; 100× objective.

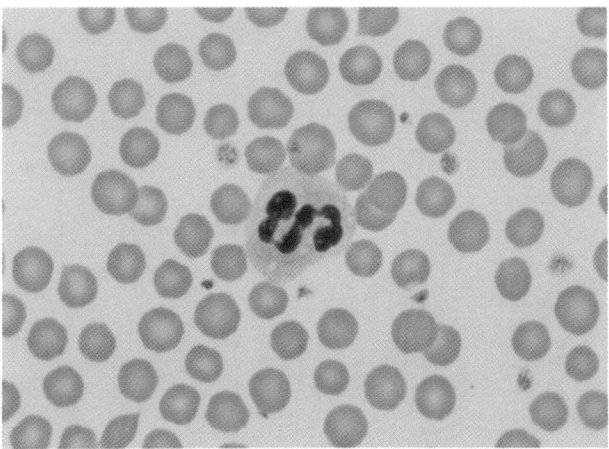

Figure 5.19. Segmented neutrophil. The cell with a segmented nucleus and light pink cytoplasm is a mature neutrophil. Bovine blood smear; 100× objective.

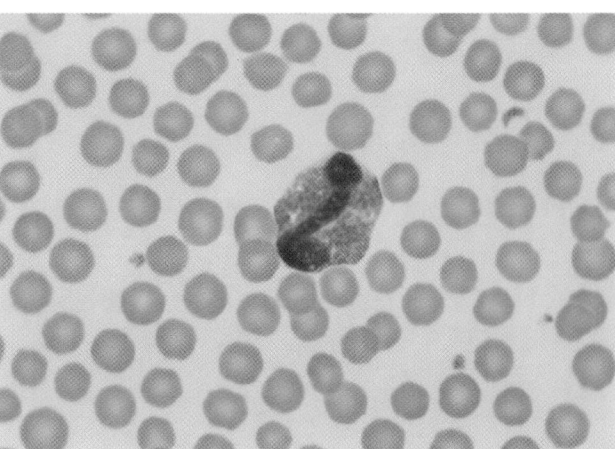

Figure 5.22. Eosinophil. The cell with the elongated nucleus and abundant, small, round reddish granules in the cytoplasm is an eosinophil. Bovine blood smear; 100× objective.

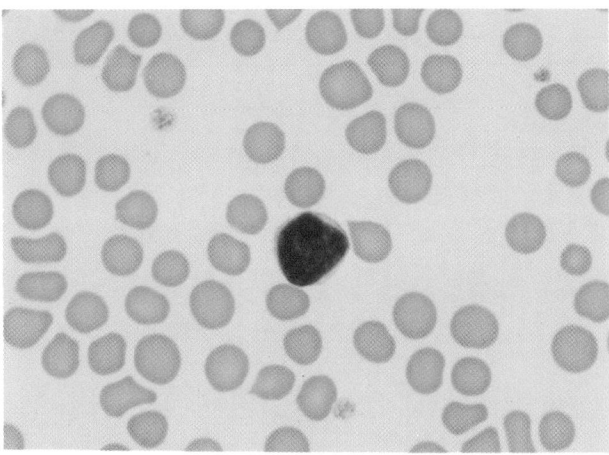

Figure 5.20. Small lymphocyte. The cell with the round to oval nucleus and a rim of light blue cytoplasm is a small lymphocyte. Bovine blood smear; 100× objective.

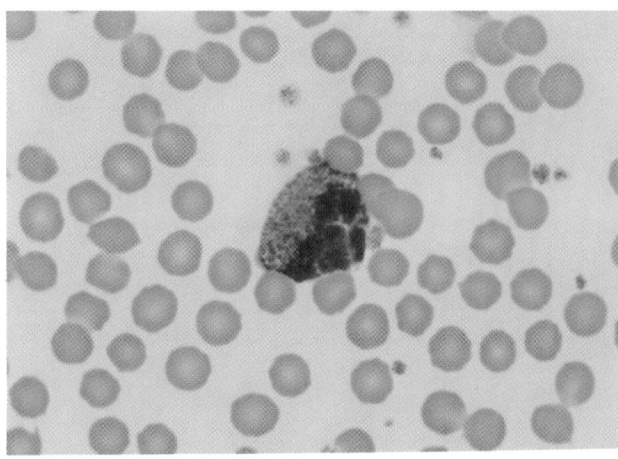

Figure 5.23. Basophil. The cell with the segmented nucleus and numerous, small purple granules in the cytoplasm is a basophil. Bovine blood smear; 100× objective.

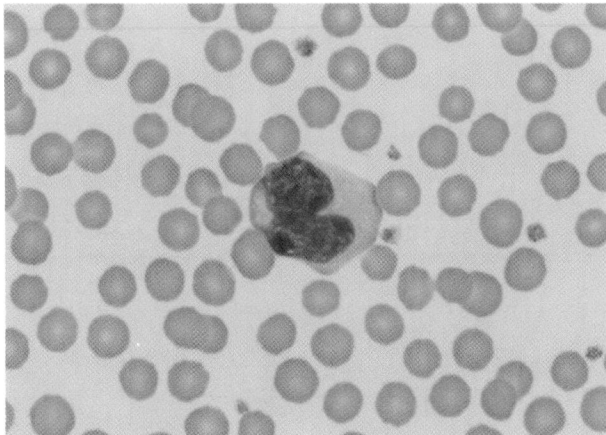

Figure 5.21. Monocyte. The large cell with the deeply indented nucleus and blue-gray cytoplasm is a monocyte. Note the lack of vacuoles, not all monocytes contain vacuoles. Bovine blood smear; 100× objective.

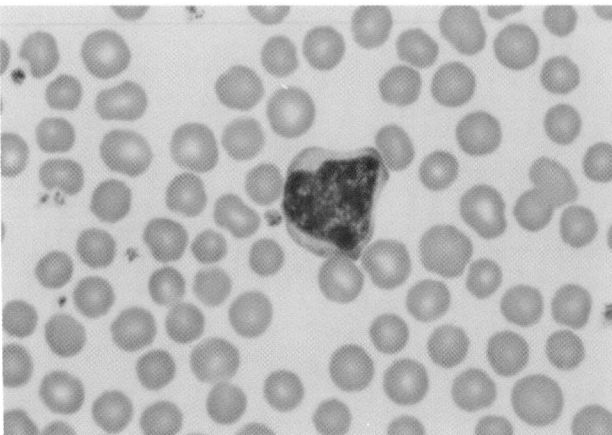

Figure 5.24. Large lymphocyte. The cell with a round to slightly indented nucleus with small amounts of light blue cytoplasm is a large lymphocyte. Note the accentuated nuclear chromatin pattern that is often seen in normal bovine lymphocytes. Bovine blood smear; 100× objective.

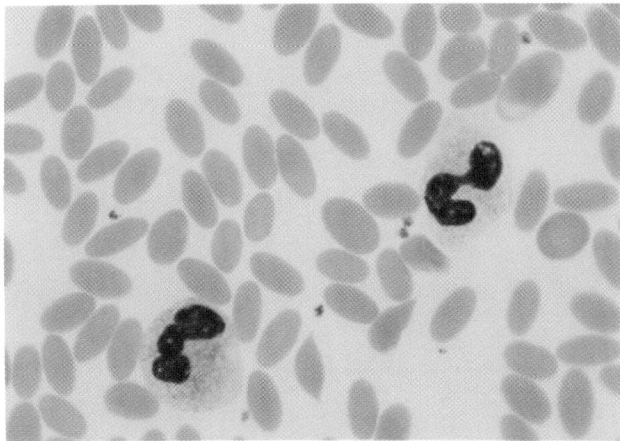

Figure 5.25. Neutrophils. The two cells with segmented nuclei and light blue to pink granular cytoplasm are segmented neutrophils. Llama blood smear; 100× objective.

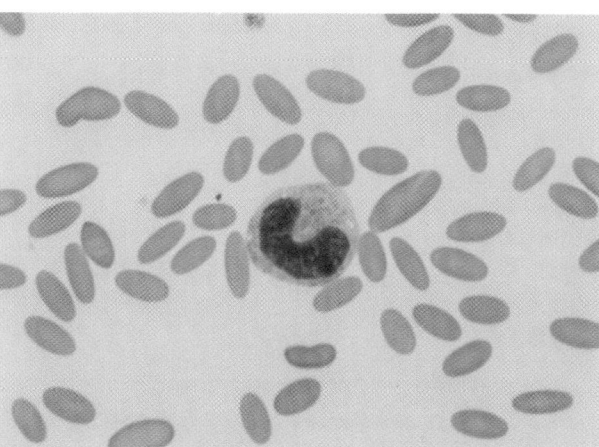

Figure 5.28. Eosinophil. The cell with a band-shaped nucleus and low numbers of poorly defined, small, round to oblong reddish granules in the cytoplasm is an eosinophil. Often llama eosinophils have low numbers of cytoplasmic granules. Llama blood smear; 100× objective.

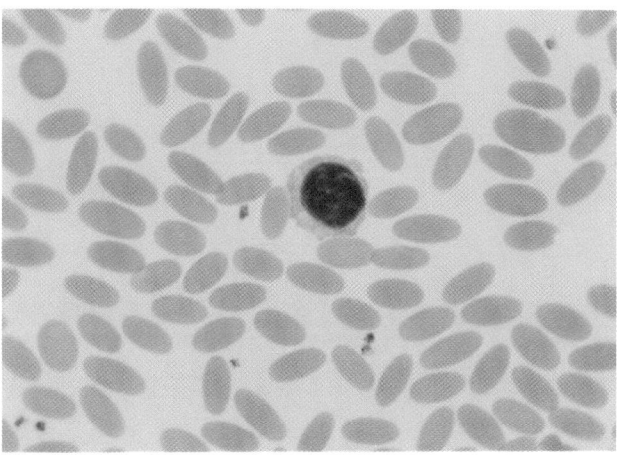

Figure 5.26. Small lymphocyte. The cell with the round nucleus and small amount of light blue cytoplasm is a small lymphocyte. Llama blood smear; 100× objective.

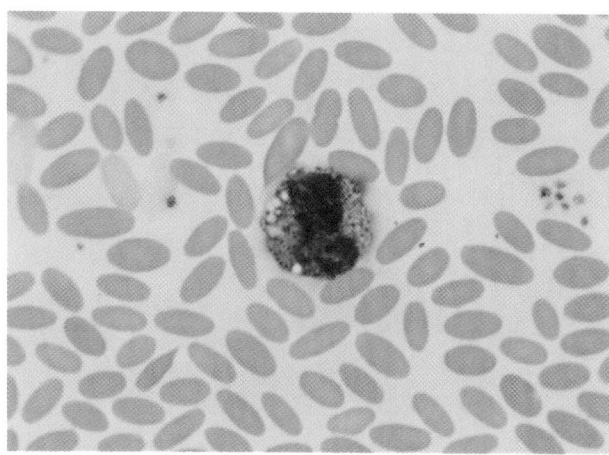

Figure 5.29. Basophil. The cell with the poorly segmented nucleus and multiple, small purple cytoplasmic granules is a basophil. The granules partially obscure the nucleus. Llama blood smear; 100× objective.

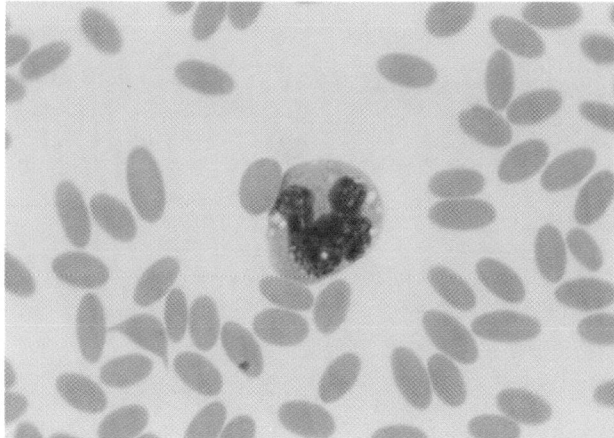

Figure 5.27. Monocyte. The large cell with a deeply indented nucleus, blue-gray cytoplasm, and multiple, discrete cytoplasmic vacuoles is a monocyte. Llama blood smear; 100× objective.

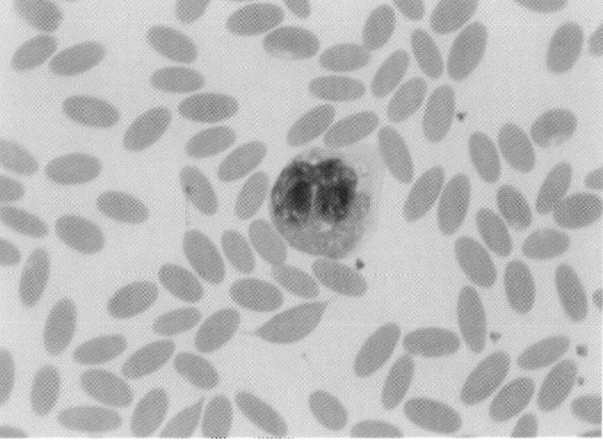

Figure 5.30. Eosinophil. The cell with a bilobed nucleus and multiple, round reddish granules is a well-granulated eosinophil. Llama blood smear; 100× objective.

CHAPTER SIX

VARIATIONS IN WHITE BLOOD CELL MORPHOLOGY

GRANULOCYTES

A common change that may be seen in animals with inflammation is the presence of increased numbers of immature neutrophilic granulocytes in the circulation. This is known as a left shift. Commonly, a left shift includes increased numbers of band neutrophils (Figure 6.1), but also may include metamyelocytes, myelocytes, and, very rarely, promyelocytes and myeloblasts. The band neutrophils, as previously described, have hyposegmented nuclei. Typically, the chromatin of the band neutrophil is less condensed than that of the mature segmented neutrophil. In contrast, in Pelger-Huët anomaly, which has been reported in dogs and cats, there is a defect that causes hyposegmentation of the granulocytes (Figure 6.2) and results in the appearance of a "false left shift." This condition is extremely rare but may be distinguished from a true left shift by the characteristics of the nuclear chromatin. In Pelger-Huët anomaly, although the cells are hyposegmented, the chromatin is very condensed as in a normally segmented neutrophil. Transient pseudo–Pelger-Huët anomaly has also been reported in some disease states.

In all domestic species during inflammation, neutrophilic granulocytes may appear in the blood with a group of morphological changes known as toxicity or toxic changes. These features are often present when there is a left shift. The three main features of toxicity that are seen include increased basophilia, foaminess, and the presence of Döhle bodies in the cytoplasm. The basophilia of the cytoplasm is due to an increased amount of ribosomal RNA (Figures 6.3–6.5). The foaminess of the cytoplasm is thought to be due to prominent lysosomes (Figures 6.6 and 6.7). The Döhle bodies are irregularly shaped, small blue-gray particles in the cytoplasm (Figure 6.8). They are lamellar aggregates of rough endoplasmic reticulum. It should be noted that Döhle bodies in cats and horses are common during inflammation and, thus, are not considered as severe a sign of toxicity as compared to the other species. Depending on the degree and cause of the inflammation, there may be one or more features of toxicity present. One cause of often severe toxicity is endotoxemia.

In addition to the three features mentioned above, another morphological change that can be seen in toxic neutrophils is toxic granulation, which is the

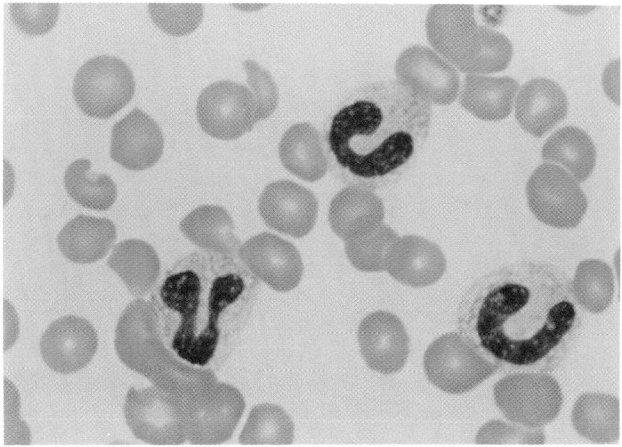

Figure 6.1. Band neutrophils. The two nucleated cells (right) are band neutrophils, and the cell in the lower left is a poorly segmented but more mature neutrophil. All these cells are toxic, based on the increased bluish color and foaminess of the cytoplasm. Canine blood smear; 100× objective.

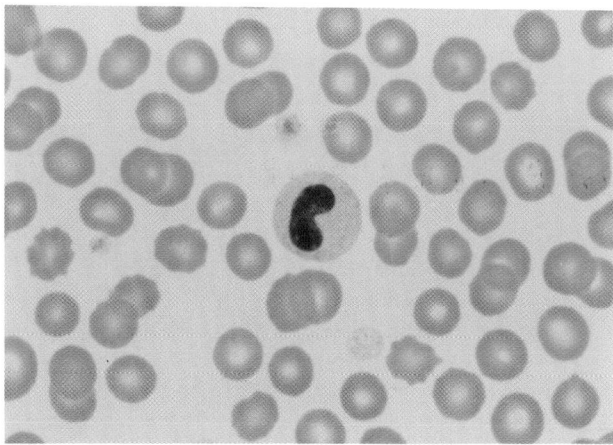

Figure 6.2. Pelger-Huët anomaly. The hyposegmented neutrophil with a very condensed chromatin pattern is typical of the Pelger-Huët anomaly. Canine blood smear; 100× objective.

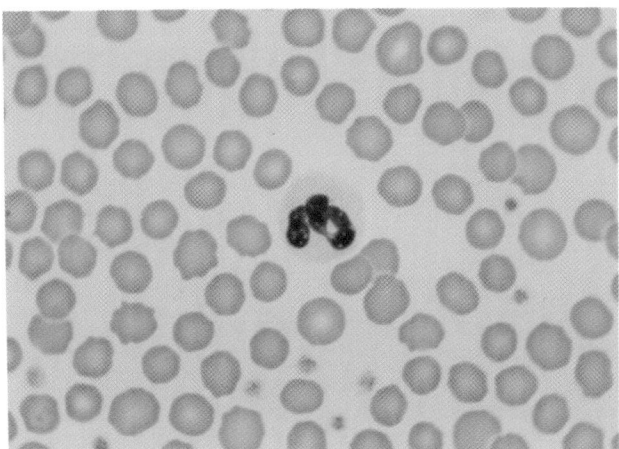

Figure 6.3. Normal segmented neutrophil. Note the light pink cytoplasm compared to the blue cytoplasm in the toxic neutrophils in Figures 6.4 and 6.5. Feline blood smear; 100× objective.

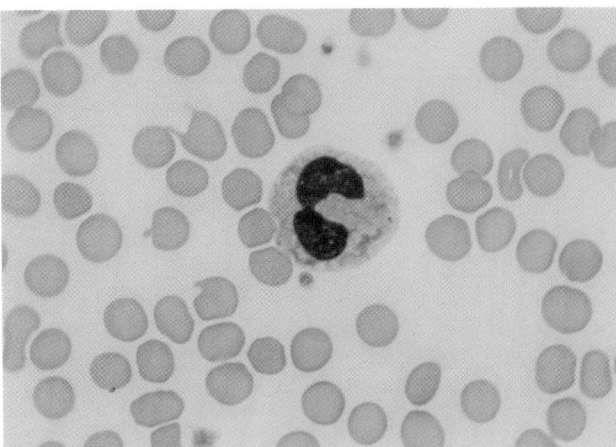

Figure 6.5. Moderate to marked cytoplasmic basophilia. The poorly segmented neutrophil in the center of the field has moderate to marked toxicity indicated by the presence of dark blue cytoplasm, foaminess of the cytoplasm, and Döhle bodies. Feline blood smear; 100× objective.

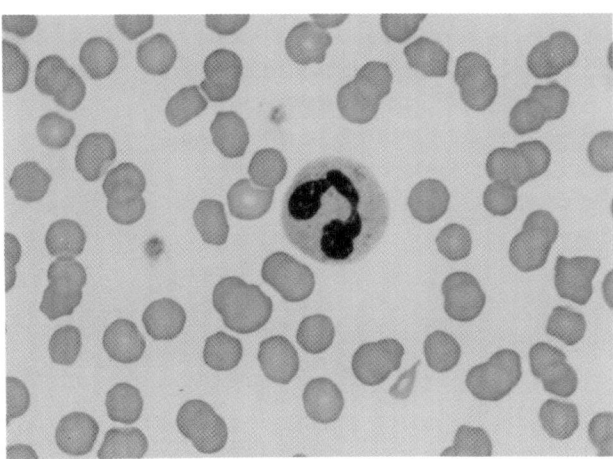

Figure 6.4. Mild to moderate cytoplasmic basophilia. The segmented neutrophil in the center of the field has mild to moderate toxicity indicated by the presence of blue cytoplasm and Döhle bodies. Feline blood smear; 100× objective.

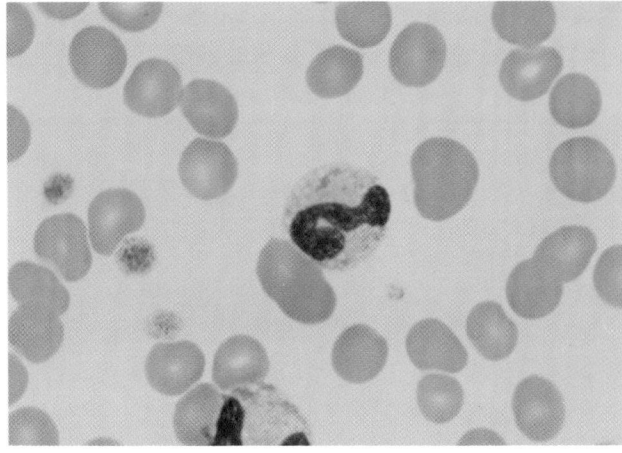

Figure 6.6. Mild cytoplasmic foaminess. There is mild foaminess of the cytoplasm of the poorly segmented neutrophil in the center of the field. Slight to moderate blue cytoplasm and Döhle bodies are also present, which further indicates moderate toxicity. Canine blood smear; 100× objective.

presence of multiple, small purple granules in the cytoplasm of the cell. These granules are probably prominent primary granules. This is not a common finding in the common domestic species but may rarely be seen in horses. Toxic granulation must be distinguished from inclusions in the neutrophils that may be seen in normal Birman cats and animals with lysosomal storage diseases.

Another rare morphological change that may be seen in animals with inflammation is the presence of giant neutrophils. These cells are produced and released more rapidly from the bone marrow, therefore the normal maturation has not occurred, thus the larger size. Giant neutrophils may also be a sign of myelodysplasia, which is described in Chapter 9.

Other miscellaneous changes that may be seen in the granulocytes are neutrophilic hypersegmentation, variably sized eosinophilic granules, and eosinophilic degranulation. Hypersegmentation may be seen in all species and is defined as neutrophils with greater than

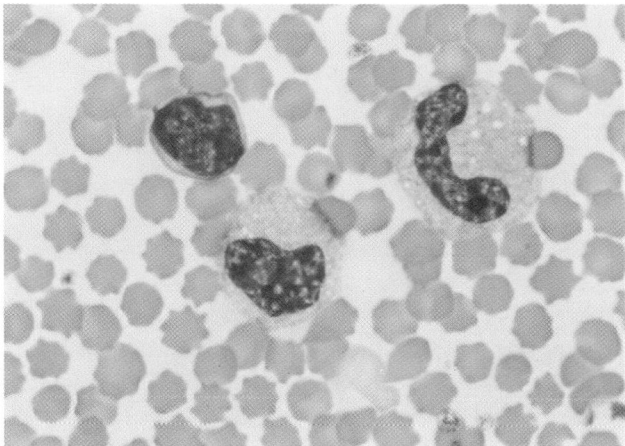

Figure 6.7. Marked cytoplasmic foaminess. The cell to the right is a band neutrophil. The cell in the center is a metamyelocyte. The cell to the left is a lymphocyte. Both the band neutrophil and metamyelocyte show signs of marked toxicity due to the marked cytoplasmic foaminess and blue cytoplasm. Bovine blood smear; 100× objective.

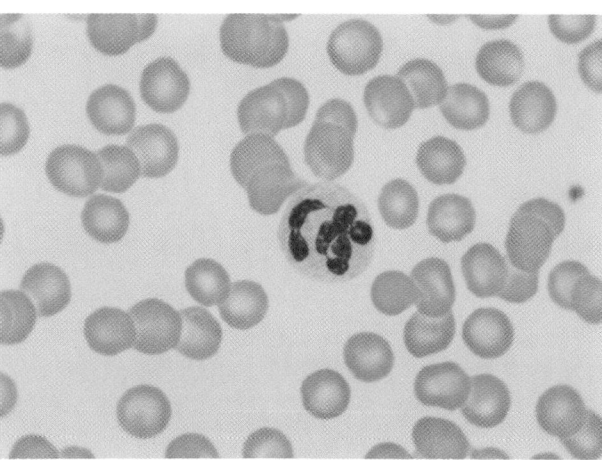

Figure 6.9. Hypersegmented neutrophil. The nucleus of the neutrophil in the center of the field has seven lobules. A cell with five or more nuclear lobules is considered hypersegmented. Canine blood smear; 100× objective.

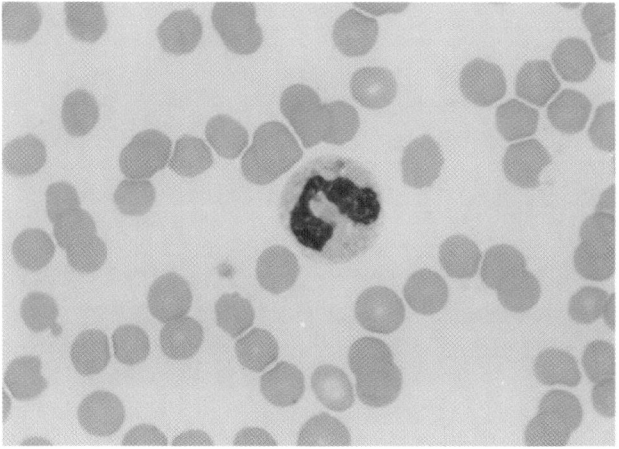

Figure 6.8. Döhle body. The irregular aggregate of blue material at the 12 o'clock position in the cytoplasm of the segmented neutrophil (center) is a Döhle body. Moderate basophilia and mild cytoplasmic foaminess are also present. Feline blood smear; 100× objective.

cells may be present with only a few larger granules and variable numbers of vacuoles.

Degranulation of the eosinophils may be seen in all species but is most recognized in dogs. Although it can occur in any breed, greyhounds often have degranulated eosinophils. These cells are often interpreted as neutrophils. The distinguishing features of degranulated eosinophils are that these cells are larger than neutrophils and often have multiple, variably sized vacuoles in the cytoplasm (Figure 6.11). Eosinophilic granules may be present in low numbers or completely absent from these cells.

5 segments or lobules (Figure 6.9). This change typically is due to the retention of the cell in the circulation much longer than normal, but it also can be seen when blood smears are not made soon enough after the blood has been collected. Hypersegmentation of the neutrophils also can occur in poodles with erythrocytic macrocytosis and giant schnauzers with B12 deficiency.

Marked variation in the size of the eosinophilic granules mainly occurs in dogs (Figure 6.10). Some

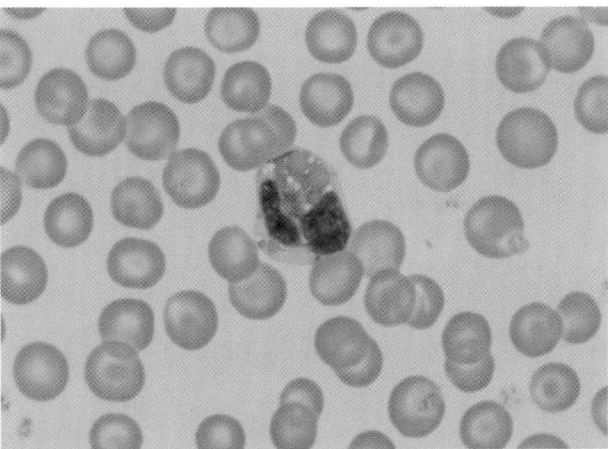

Figure 6.10. Eosinophil with large, variably sized granules. The nucleated cell (center) is an eosinophil with large, variably sized, reddish granules. Canine blood smear; 100× objective.

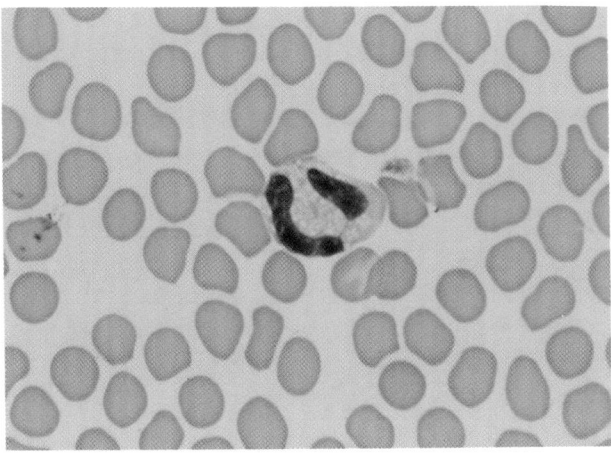

Figure 6.11. Degranulated eosinophil. The cell in the center of the field with a bilobed nucleus joined by a thin filament and multiple, variably sized, poorly defined vacuoles is a degranulated greyhound eosinophil. Canine blood smear; 100× objective.

AGRANULOCYTES

The major different morphological changes that occur in the agranulocytes are variations in morphology of lymphocytes. Reactive lymphocytes, also known as immunocytes, are typically lymphocytes with dark blue cytoplasm and possibly increased amounts of cytoplasm (Figures 6.12–6.14). These cells may also have a prominent perinuclear clear zone. Low numbers of reactive lymphocytes can be found in normal animals but typically are found in increased numbers in animals that are antigenically stimulated.

Plasma cells or plasmacytoid reactive lymphocytes are rarely seen in the peripheral blood. These cells have much more cytoplasm than normal or reactive lymphocytes. The cytoplasm is deep blue to blue-green. Often there is a prominent perinuclear clear zone. The nucleus is round with marked condensation of the chromatin in some areas and clear in other areas. Rarely, these cells may have multiple discrete vacuoles in the cytoplasm that are known as Russell bodies.

Atypical lymphocyte is a term that is used differently by different people. We describe atypical lymphocytes as those cells with morphology similar to that of reactive lymphocytes, but in addition to dark blue cytoplasm and possibly increased amounts of cytoplasm, there are nuclear abnormalities. In contrast to normal lymphocytes where the nucleus is round to slightly indented, the nucleus of atypical lymphocytes has deep clefts and/or multiple indentations or infoldings (Figure 6.15). The presence of a rare atypical lymphocyte may be associated with just antigenic stimulation. However, the presence of high numbers of these cells may indicate that the animal has a lymphoproliferative disorder (see Chapter 9).

Lymphoblasts are lymphocytes with nuclei that contain one or more nucleoli (Figure 6.16). These cells typically are much larger than small lymphocytes, although small lymphoblasts may be seen. The nucleus of a lymphoblast not only contains a prominent nucleolus, but the chromatin also is more open and finely stippled compared to that of the normal small lymphocyte. If lymphoblasts are easy to find in the peripheral blood, the animal most likely has a lymphoproliferative disorder. Due to the marked accentuation of the chromatin of the normal bovine large lymphocyte, these cells are often misinterpreted as lymphoblasts.

Normal monocytic morphology has been previously described. The major variation in monocytic morphology is that some monocytes lack prominent vacuoles (Figures 6.17 and 6.18). This can occur in any

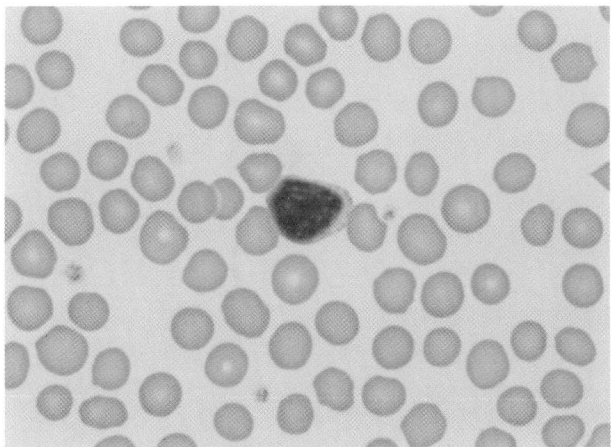

Figure 6.12. Normal small lymphocyte. Note the light blue cytoplasm compared to the dark blue cytoplasm of the reactive lymphocytes in Figures 6.12 and 6.13. Feline blood smear; 100× objective.

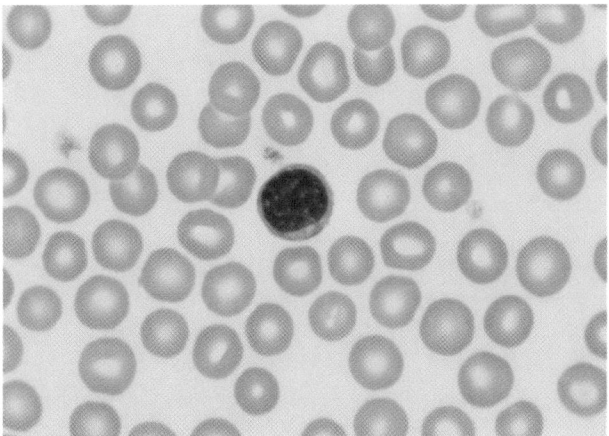

Figure 6.13. Reactive lymphocyte. The dark blue cytoplasm and poorly defined, perinuclear clear zone are typical of a reactive lymphocyte. Canine blood smear; 100× objective.

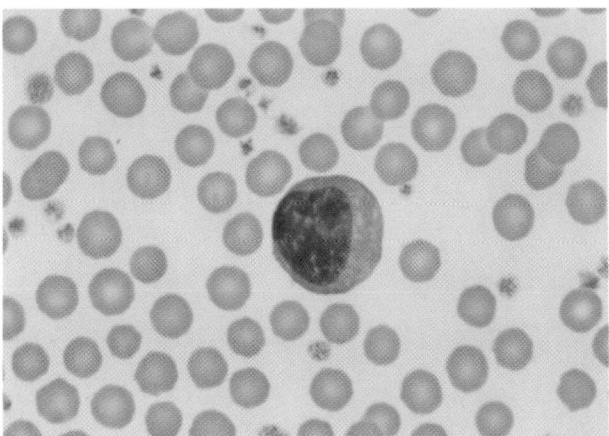

Figure 6.14. Reactive lymphocyte. This lymphocyte has increased amounts of dark blue cytoplasm, which is supportive of reactivity. Bovine blood smear; 100× objective.

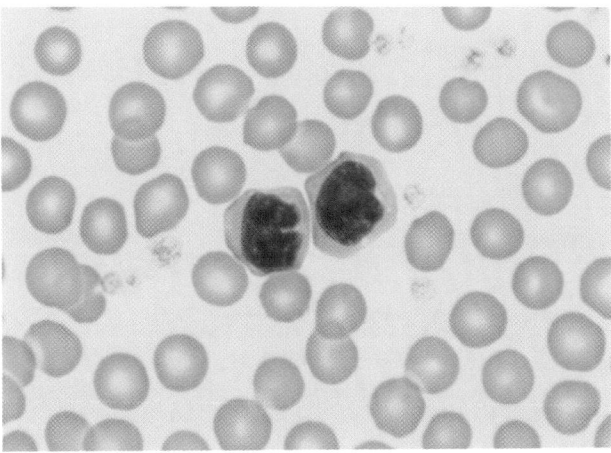

Figure 6.15. Atypical lymphocytes. The two cells (center) with deeply clefted nuclei and dark blue cytoplasm are atypical lymphocytes. This animal had a lymphoproliferative disorder, based on the presence of high numbers of lymphocytes and atypical morphology. Canine blood smear; 100× objective.

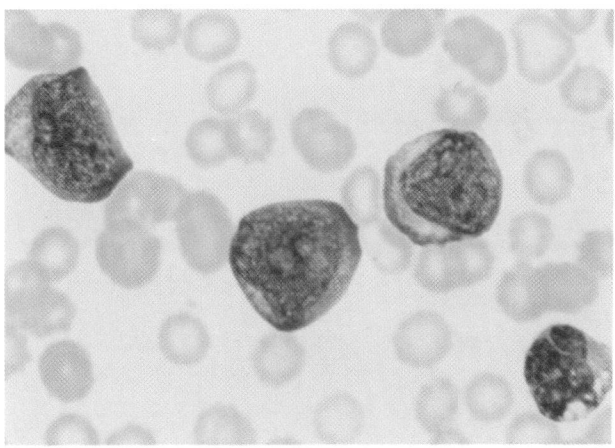

Figure 6.16. Lymphoblasts. The three largest cells with round to oval nuclei, single or multiple nucleoli, and small amounts of blue cytoplasm are lymphoblasts. Canine blood smear; 100× objective.

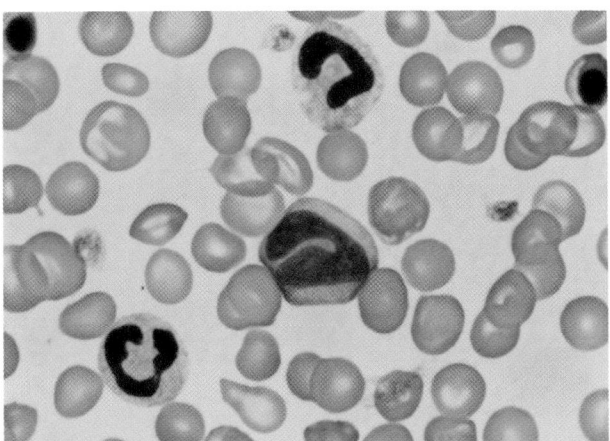

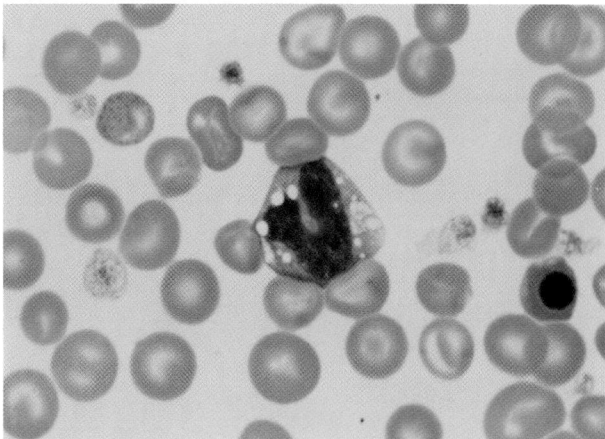

Figure 6.17. Monocyte. The large cell (center) with a deeply indented nucleus and blue-gray cytoplasm with no cytoplasmic vacuoles is a monocyte. Note the pale, finely granular nuclear chromatin compared with the condensed chromatin of the toxic band neutrophil (top center). There is also a toxic segmented neutrophil present (lower left) and metarubricytes (top left and right corners). Canine blood smear; 100× objective.

Figure 6.18. Monocyte. The large cell (center) with a deeply indented nucleus and blue-gray cytoplasm is a monocyte. Note the multiple, discrete, clear cytoplasmic vacuoles in the monocyte compared with the monocyte in Figure 6.17; these photomicrographs are from the same blood smear. A metarubricyte is present (lower right) and a red blood cell with basophilic stippling is present (upper left). Canine blood smear; 100× objective.

species. When these cells lack vacuoles, they may be confused with band neutrophils or atypical lymphocytes. Usually, if there is any question in interpretation, more-typical monocytes with vacuoles can be found on the blood smear, and these cells can be use-ful in confirming that the cells without vacuoles are truly monocytes. Also, the chromatin of the monocyte is more granular to lacy with some areas of condensation compared to the more condensed chromatin of the band neutrophil.

CHAPTER SEVEN

WHITE BLOOD CELL INCLUSIONS AND PARASITES

Overall, the presence of inclusions or parasites in white blood cells is a much less common finding than inclusions or parasites in red blood cells. Also, if inclusions or parasites are present, they are often present in extremely low numbers.

Azurophilic granules, which may be confused with viral inclusions or parasites, are present in some normal lymphocytes. These typically small, variably sized, and often multiple pink to purple granules can be found in lymphocytes of any species (Figure 7.1). Rarely, these granules can be quite large, especially in ruminants. In most normal animals, only a small percentage of lymphocytes are granulated. In the llama, a fairly high proportion of normal lymphocytes has been reported to have these granules.

Organisms can be found in the white blood cells of dogs with ehrlichiosis. The *Ehrlichia* morulae can be a few to several microns in diameter. Each morula is made up of multiple, small, blue to purple coccoid-shaped structures known as elementary bodies. When morulae are present in monocytes or lymphocytes, they are typically *Ehrlichia canis*, found mainly in tropical and subtropical areas. Morulae that are present in neutrophils or eosinophils are typically *Ehrlichia ewingii* (Figure 7.2). This form of ehrlichiosis is known as granulocytic ehrlichiosis.

Distemper viral inclusions in dogs can potentially be found in all types of white blood cells. They are quite variable in size and stain pink to light purple. These round, oval to oblong, irregular structures have a granular to often a smooth glassy appearance (Figure 7.3). Single or multiple inclusions may be present.

Hepatozoon canis is typically found in the neutrophils or monocytes. Cases have been mainly reported in the U.S. Gulf Coast states, France, Italy, the

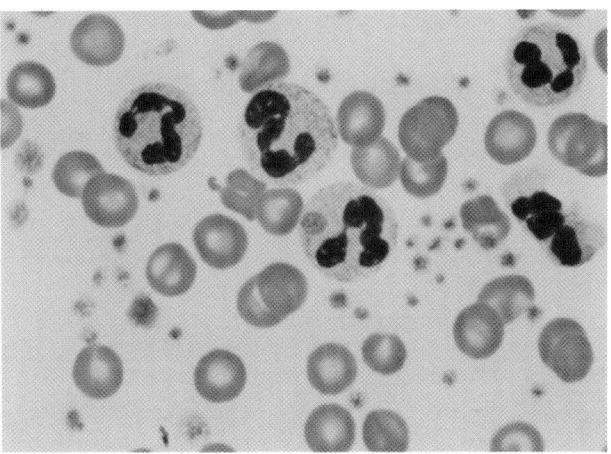

Figure 7.2. Morula of *Ehrlichia ewingii*. The neutrophil in the center of the field has a single cytoplasmic morula. Canine buffy coat smear, courtesy of D. Boon; 100× objective.

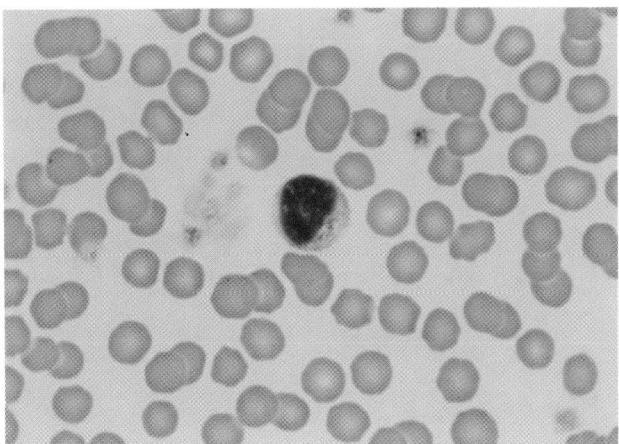

Figure 7.1. Azurophilic granules. The lymphocyte has several small, pink to purple cytoplasmic granules adjacent to the nucleus. Feline blood smear; 100× objective.

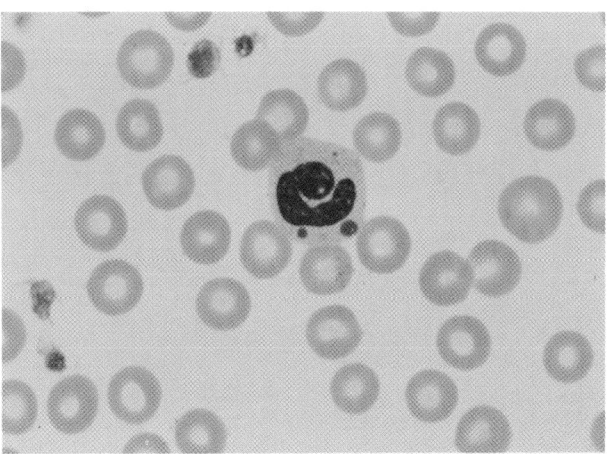

Figure 7.3. Canine distemper viral inclusions. The segmented neutrophil in the center of the field has prominent, round, light purple cytoplasmic inclusions characteristic of canine distemper virus. Canine blood smear; 100× objective.

43

Middle East, and Asia. *H. canis* gametocytes are large, oblong to oval organisms, typically measuring 5 × 10 μm and stain light blue (Figure 7.4).

Histoplasma capsulatum can be found in neutrophils, monocytes, and eosinophils in the United States and sporadically elsewhere. They are 2 to 4 μm in diameter, round to oval structures (Figure 7.5). They stain light blue and contain pink to purple, eccentrically placed granular nuclear material. Often there is a small halo around the organism. Single or multiple organisms may be present.

Mucopolysaccharidoses are a group of uncommon lysosomal storage diseases in cats as well as dogs. Mucopolysaccharidoses types I, VI, and VII in cats and type VII in dogs have been reported to have pinpoint purple granules in the cytoplasm of neutrophils (Figure 7.6). Cats with GM$_2$ gangliosidosis, another lysosomal storage disease, also have neutrophil granulation. Granulation may be seen in other white blood cell types in these disorders as well. Granulation of the lysosomal storage disease can look similar to toxic granulation and may be distinguished from it because there are typically no other signs of toxicity in the neutrophils. Biochemical testing is required to confirm the type of lysosomal storage disease. Similar granulation has been seen in neutrophils in some Birman cats. These cats do not have clinical signs that are typically associated with lysosomal storage diseases.

Certain types of lysosomal storage diseases in cats, including Nieman-Pick disease, gangliosidosis, mucopolysaccharidosis, and mannosidosis, result in vacuolation of white blood cells. These multiple, small discrete vacuoles are most easily recognized in lymphocytes (Figure 7.7). In some of these storage diseases, granules may also be found inside a portion of the vacuoles. Biochemical characterization of the enzyme deficiency is necessary to confirm and accurately classify the disorder. Fresh blood smears should be examined since vacuolation of normal white blood cells may also occur over time in vitro. Vacuolation of neutrophils has also been reported in cats after administration of high doses of chloramphenicol and phenylbutazone.

Another rare hereditary disorder of cats in which

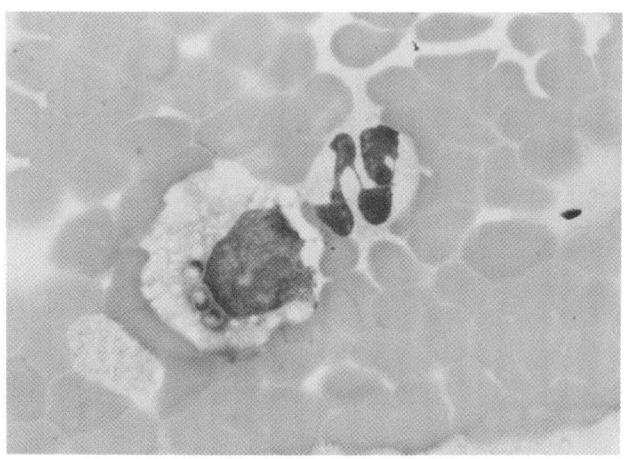

Figure 7.5. *Histoplasma capsulatum.* The monocyte/macrophage has three light blue oval organisms with purple, eccentrically placed granular material. These are *Histoplasma capsulatum* organisms. Canine blood smear, feathered edge; 100× objective.

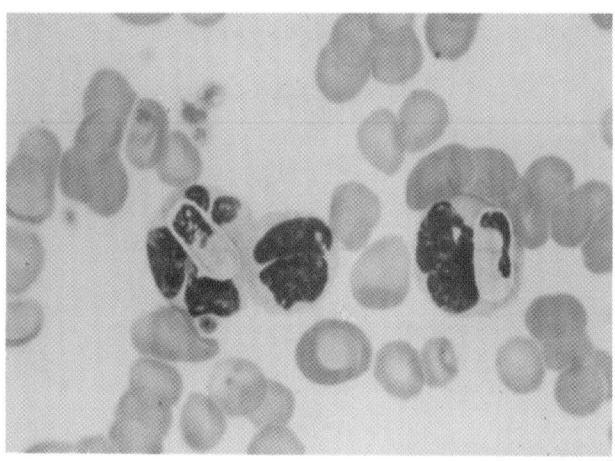

Figure 7.4. *Hepatozoon canis.* Two of three neutrophils in the center of the field have single, large, oblong cytoplasmic structures with eccentrically placed, purple granular material. These are gametocytes of *Hepatozoon canis*. Canine blood smear; 100× objective.

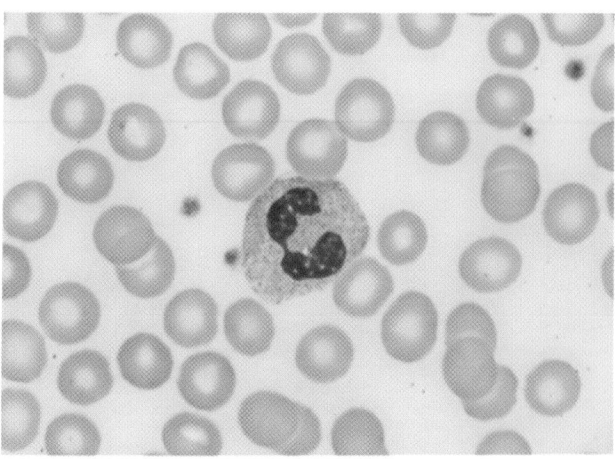

Figure 7.6. Mucopolysaccharidosis type VI. The neutrophil in the center of the field has multiple, small, light purple granules in the cytoplasm; this is typical of mucopolysaccharidosis type VI. Feline blood smear; 100× objective.

leukocyte inclusions may be present is Chédiak-Higashi syndrome (Figure 7.8). The granules are typically round to oval, 2 μm in diameter to slightly larger. They stain light pink, and single or multiple granules may be present.

Inclusions and parasites in white blood cells of horses are uncommon. *Ehrlichia equi* (mainly U.S.A.) looks similar to *Ehrlichia canis* and can be found in neutrophils and rarely in eosinophils.

Inclusions and parasites in white blood cells of cattle are also uncommon. *Ehrlichia phagocytophilia* is re-

ported in Northern and Western Europe. The rare hereditary disorder, Chédiak-Higashi syndrome, has been reported in cattle and looks similar to the inclusions described for cats.

Vacuolation of cow as well as sheep lymphocytes has been reported in the lysosomal storage disease known as acquired alpha mannosidosis. The decrease in the enzyme activity of alpha mannosidase is due to the ingestion of swainsonine, which is found in the locoweed plant. Measurement of swainsonine in the blood can be done to confirm this disease.

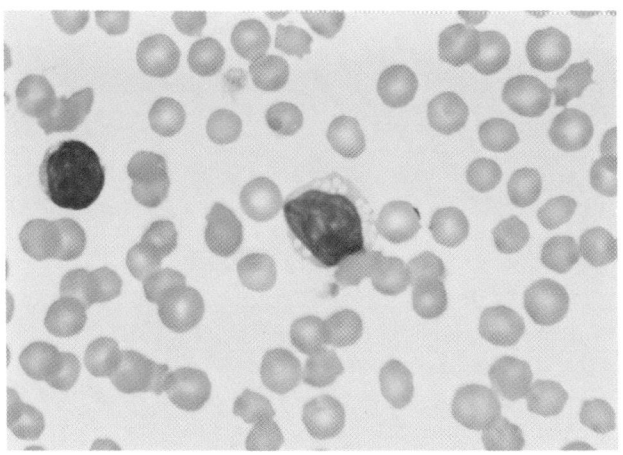

Figure 7.7. Gangliosidosis. The lymphocyte in the center of the field has multiple, variably sized, discrete cytoplasmic vacuoles typical of some lysosomal storage diseases, including gangliosidosis. The lymphocyte to the left is more normal appearing. Feline blood smear, from 1988 ASVCP slide review, courtesy of S. Dial; 100× objective.

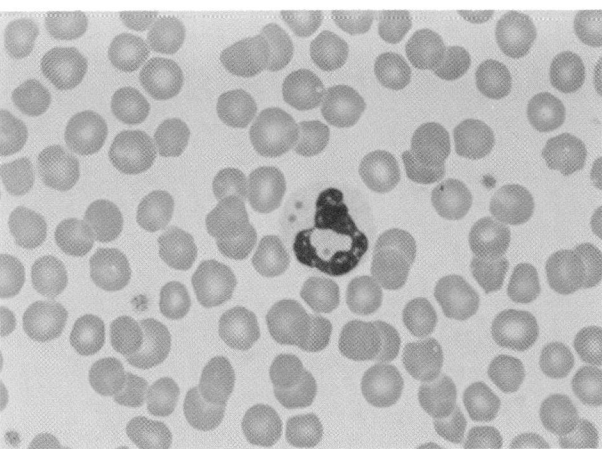

Figure 7.8. Chédiak-Higashi syndrome. The neutrophil in the center of the field has three small, round, pink cytoplasmic granules typical of Chédiak-Higashi syndrome. Feline blood smear, from 1987 ASVCP slide review, courtesy of M. Menard; 100× objective.

CHAPTER EIGHT
PLATELETS

Platelets, also known as thrombocytes, morphologically look very similar in the different species, although in horses they generally do not stain as intensely (Figures 8.1–8.5). Platelets are small, anucleated, discoid-shaped, light blue staining cells that may have multiple, fine, pink to purple granules in the cytoplasm. They are typically 2 to 4 μm in diameter. Sometimes, if platelets become activated during the collection procedure, they may have multiple fine projections. If enough of the platelets are activated, they will coalesce and form large clumps (Figure 8.6). It is sometimes difficult to make out the individual platelets in these clumps. Often due to their large size, platelet clumps can be found on the feathered edge of the slide.

With increased demand for platelets, larger platelets may be released from the bone marrow. These larger platelets are known as macroplatelets or giant platelets (Figure 8.7). These platelets typically can be 5 μm or larger. Macroplatelets are commonly seen in feline peripheral blood samples irrespective of disease state; in this species, this finding is not necessarily related to bone marrow response to a peripheral demand for platelets.

A rickettsial organism that has an affinity for platelets is *Ehrlichia platys*. Infection by this organism causes a disease that occurs in dogs mainly in the southern and southeastern portions of the United States and elsewhere in tropical and subtropical areas. The morphology of these organisms is similar to that of the *Ehrlichia* species that infects white blood cells. The morulae are a few microns in diameter and are made up of multiple, small, blue to purple coccoid-shaped structures known as elementary bodies (Figure 8.8).

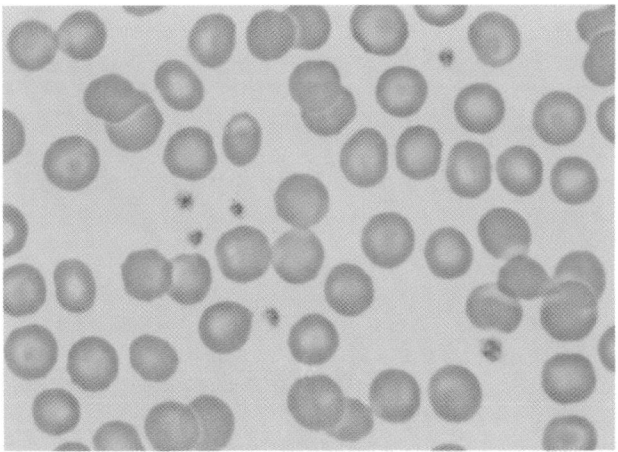

Figure 8.1. Dog platelets. The small, round to oval, light blue anucleated cells with pink to purple cytoplasmic granules are platelets. Canine blood smear; 100× objective.

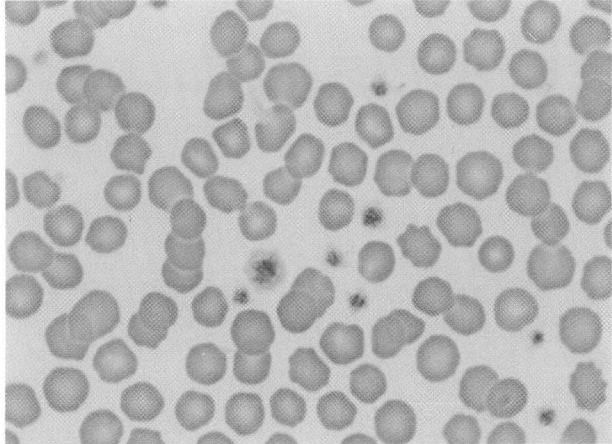

Figure 8.2. Cat platelets. The small, round to oval, light blue anucleated cells with pink to purple cytoplasmic granules are platelets. Note the larger size of some of the platelets that are common in cats. Feline blood smear; 100× objective.

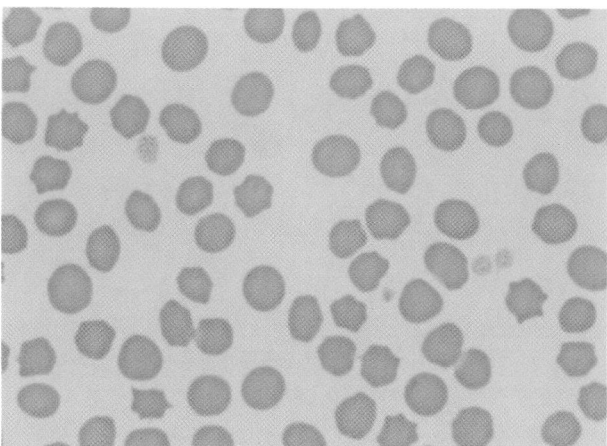

Figure 8.3. Horse platelets. The small, round to oval, very light blue anucleated cells with indistinct, pink cytoplasmic granules are platelets. These cells typically do not stain as intensely in horses as they do in other species. Equine blood smear; 100× objective.

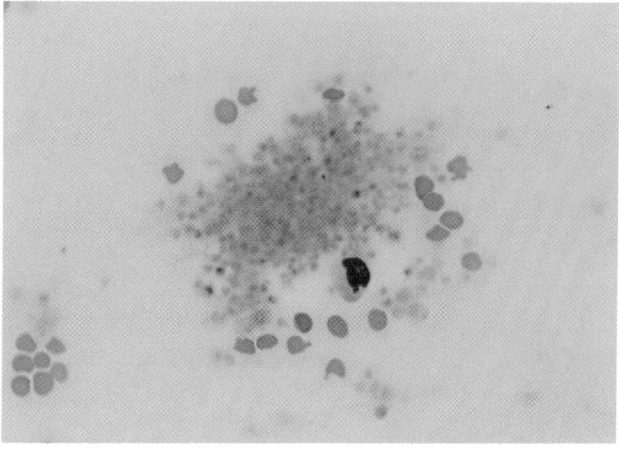

Figure 8.6. Large platelet clump. A large irregular clump of platelets is present (center). Note the size of the platelet clump compared with the neutrophil that is also present. Feline blood smear, feathered edge; 50× objective.

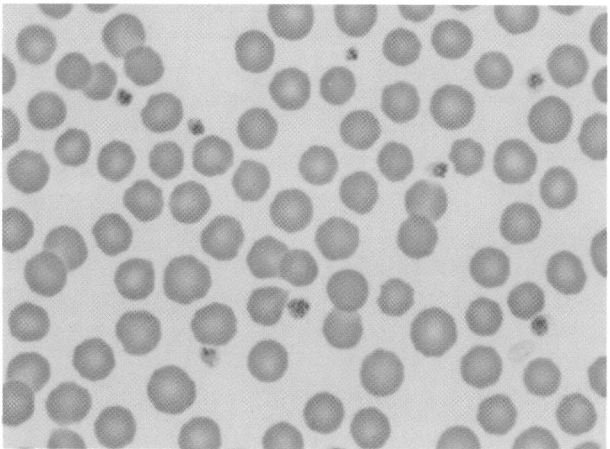

Figure 8.4. Cow platelets. The small, round to oval, light blue anucleated cells with pink to purple cytoplasmic granules are platelets. Bovine blood smear; 100× objective.

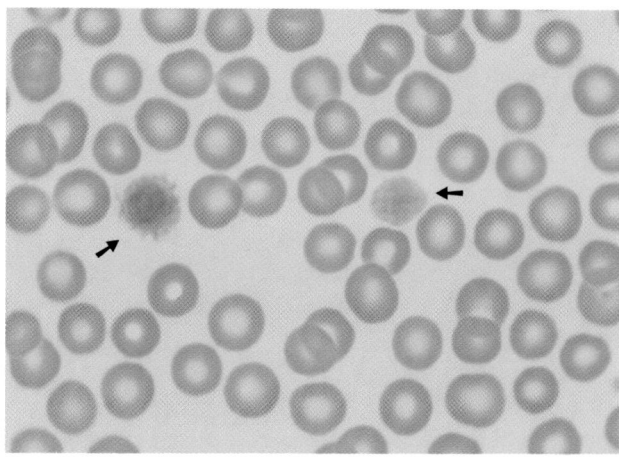

Figure 8.7. Macroplatelets. Two giant, or macro-, platelets are present (arrows). Canine blood smear; 100× objective.

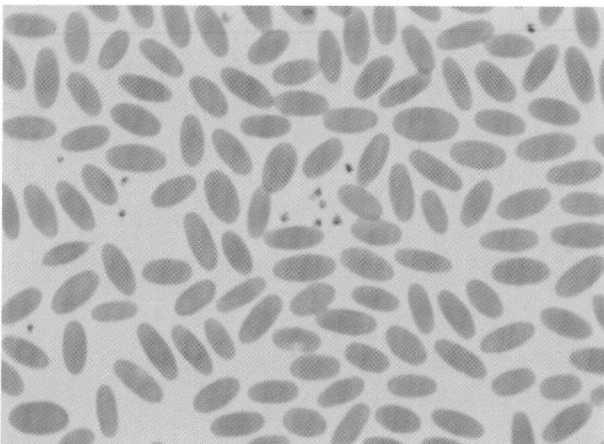

Figure 8.5. Llama platelets. The very small, round to oval, light blue anucleated cells with pink to purple cytoplasmic granules are platelets. Llama blood smear; 100× objective.

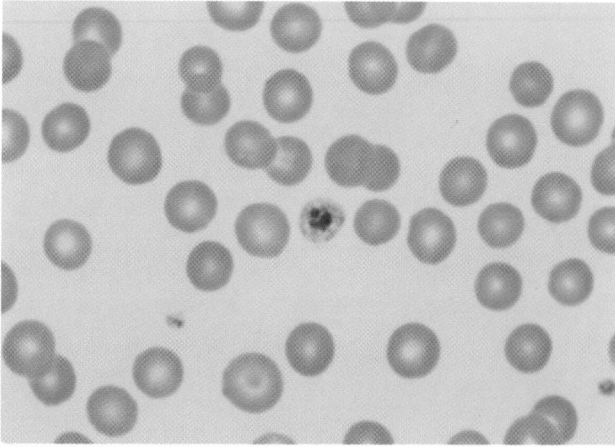

Figure 8.8. *Ehrlichia platys.* The large platelet in the center of the field has two small, dark purple inclusions that are morulae of *Ehrlichia platys.* Canine blood smear, from 1986 ASVCP slide review, courtesy of S. Gaunt; 100× objective.

CHAPTER NINE

LYMPHOPROLIFERATIVE AND MYELOPROLIFERATIVE DISORDERS

GENERAL FEATURES

Animals with lymphoproliferative or myeloproliferative disorders have clonal proliferation of neoplastic cells of the lymphoid and myeloid lineage respectively. When this neoplastic proliferation occurs in the bone marrow and these cells are released into the circulation, this is known as leukemia. The diagnosis of leukemia depends on several different factors, including history, clinical signs, and physical examination, as well as a detailed examination of the blood and bone marrow.

Recently, the animal leukemia study group of the American Society of Veterinary Clinical Pathologists (ASVCP) proposed the adaptation of the French/American/British classification scheme of leukemias of people to be used in the classification of myeloid leukemias of dogs and cats. This system is based on recognizing the abnormal cells that are present, as well as systematically counting the different cell types present in the bone marrow. This classification scheme, although very useful, is beyond the scope of this atlas and is not used extensively here. Instead, the basic morphological approach is given for both lymphoid and myeloid leukemia. The discussion in this chapter focuses on those changes that are present in the peripheral blood of animals with leukemia, but again, this clearly is only one factor to consider in recognizing and classifying leukemias.

Finding an abnormality in the peripheral blood is often the first indication that a leukemia may be present. With poorly differentiated leukemia, identification of a leukemic process is often easy; the difficulty lies in the proper classification. It is common in these cases to use special enzyme cytochemical stains or immunophenotyping to properly identify the origin of the neoplastic cells. In contrast, in well-differentiated leukemia, the cell lineage is easy to recognize, but the challenge is to differentiate the leukemic process from inflammation.

LYMPHOPROLIFERATIVE DISORDERS

Lymphocytic Leukemia

Lymphocytic leukemia can occur in any species but is more common in dogs and cats compared to horses, cattle, and llamas. Lymphocytic leukemia can be divided into two major types: acute and chronic.

Acute Lymphocytic Leukemia Animals with acute lymphocytic leukemia, also known as acute lymphoblastic leukemia, often have high numbers of neoplastic cells in the circulation, but the morphology of these lymphocytes is not typical of those found in the circulation of a normal animal. In acute lymphocytic leukemia, the predominant cell type is a large, immature-appearing lymphocyte, typically a lymphoblast (Figures 9.1 and 9.2).

Chronic Lymphocytic Leukemia In chronic lymphocytic leukemia, the predominant cell type is a cytomorphologically normal lymphocyte. These lymphocytes usually look similar to typical small- to medium-sized lymphocytes present in the circulation, but they are present in very high numbers (Figures 9.3 and 9.4).

Lymphosarcoma

Lymphoblasts also may be found in the circulation during the leukemic phase of lymphosarcoma (Figure 9.5). Lymphosarcoma is a lymphoproliferative disorder in which, typically, the neoplastic lymphocyte proliferation starts in primary sites other than the bone marrow, such as lymph nodes and tissues. In certain cases, the proliferation of the neoplastic cells will spread to the bone marrow and subsequently to the blood, leading to the leukemic phase of lymphosarcoma. Because of the higher incidence of lymphosarcoma than acute lymphocytic leukemia, circulating lymphoblasts are more commonly seen with lymphosarcoma.

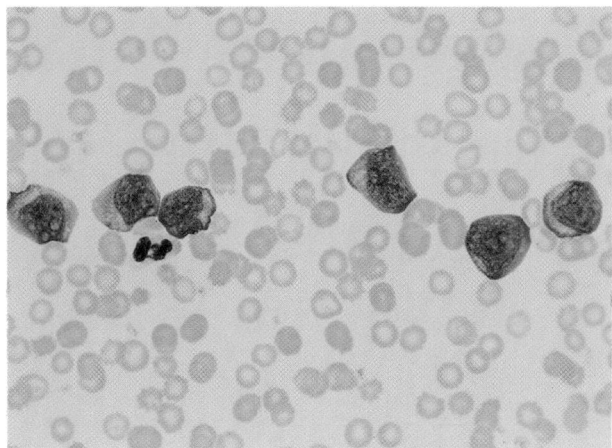

Figure 9.1. Acute lymphocytic leukemia. Many large lymphocytes, often with prominent nucleoli, are present. Note the large size of these cells relative to the normal neutrophil in the left center of the field. Canine blood smear; 50× objective.

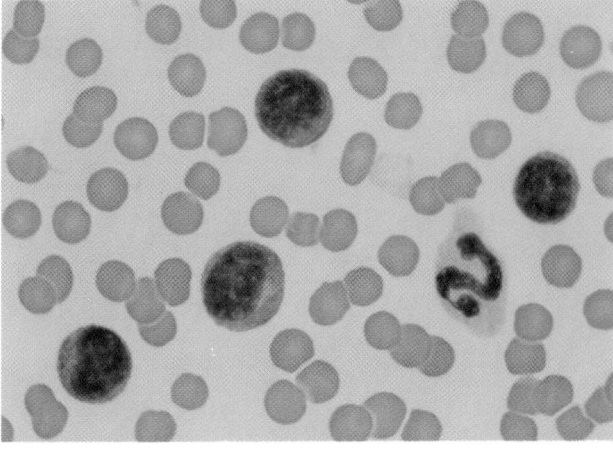

Figure 9.4. Chronic lymphocytic leukemia. This is a higher magnification of the blood smear shown in Figure 9.3. Note the four small- to medium-sized lymphocytes that are normal to slightly reactive in morphology. Feline blood smear; 100× objective.

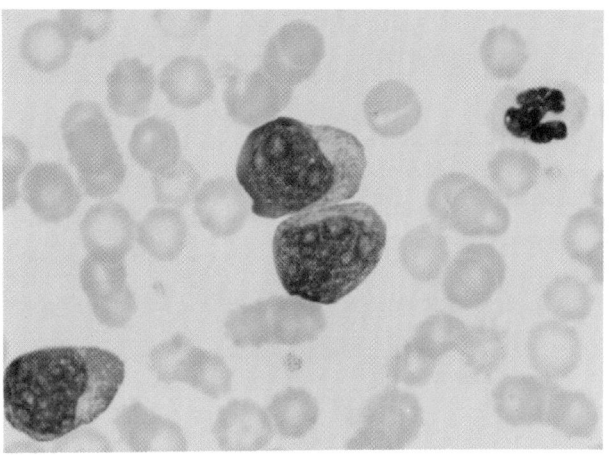

Figure 9.2. Acute lymphocytic leukemia. This is a higher magnification of the blood smear shown in Figure 9.1. Three large lymphocytes are present with prominent multiple nucleoli; these are lymphoblasts. A normal neutrophil is present in the upper right corner. Canine blood smear; 100× objective.

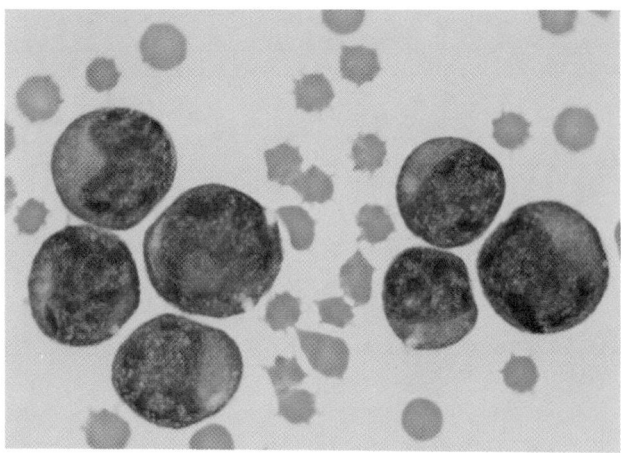

Figure 9.5. Lymphoblasts. Seven large lymphocytes are present, often with prominent nucleoli; these are lymphoblasts. This animal is in the leukemic phase of lymphosarcoma. Bovine blood smear; 100× objective.

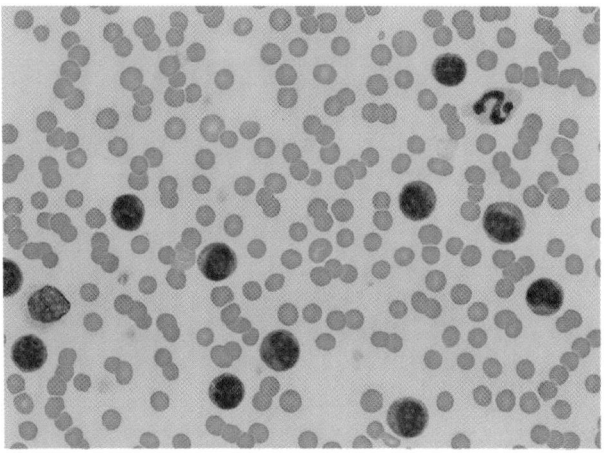

Figure 9.3. Chronic lymphocytic leukemia. Many small- to medium-sized lymphocytes are present in this field. One segmented neutrophil is in the upper right corner. Feline blood smear; 50× objective.

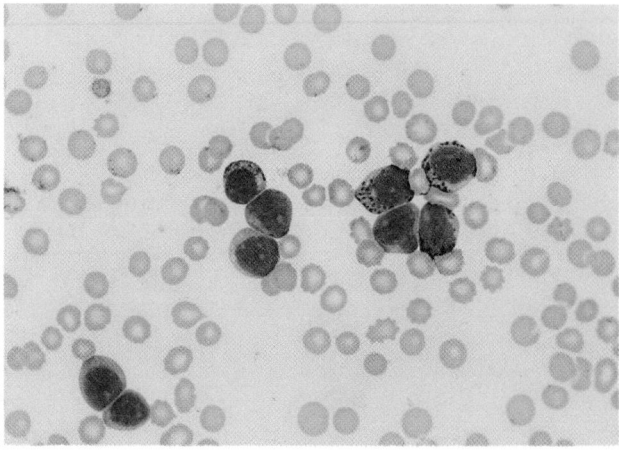

Figure 9.6. Large granular lymphocytic leukemia. Many large lymphocytes, often with prominent nucleoli, are present. Several of the cells also have large, round to irregularly shaped, purple cytoplasmic granules. Canine blood smear, from 1989 ASVCP slide review, courtesy of M. Wellman; 50× objective.

Large Granular Lymphocytic Leukemia

Another rare lymphoproliferative disorder that is unique due to the morphology of the lymphocytes is large granular lymphocytic leukemia (Figures 9.6 and 9.7). As the name implies, these cells have large, variably sized, purple cytoplasmic granules.

Plasma Cell Myeloma

Finally, a lymphoproliferative disorder in which the neoplastic proliferation mainly occurs in the bone marrow is plasma cell myeloma. Plasma cells rarely can be seen in the circulation with this disorder. Plasma cells are not typically found in the circulation in animals with inflammatory disease, thus if present in high numbers, plasma cell myeloma should be considered.

MYELOPROLIFERATIVE DISORDERS

General Features

As with lymphoproliferative disorders, myeloproliferative disorders are more common in small animals than in large animals. These disorders are most commonly recognized in cats and are often associated with feline leukemia virus infection. Myeloproliferative disorders involve cells of the granulocytic, monocytic, erythrocytic, and megakaryocytic lineages. Myeloproliferative disorders can be divided into three main categories: myelodysplastic syndrome, acute myeloid leukemia, and chronic myeloid leukemia. Myeloid leukemia can be a neoplastic proliferation of cells of single, as well as multiple, lineages.

Myelodysplastic Syndrome

Myelodysplastic syndrome is most often seen in cats. Myelodysplastic syndrome is also known as preleukemia, for animals with myelodysplastic syndrome may go on to develop myeloid leukemia. Although all animals with myelodysplastic syndrome will not progress to blatant leukemia, it is still a life-threatening condition. As with leukemia, the diagnosis of myelodysplastic syndrome depends on multiple factors including history, clinical signs, physical examination, as well as a detailed examination of the blood and bone marrow; repeated examination of the blood, over time, is often necessary. Animals with myelodysplastic syndrome have abnormalities in the maturation of one or more myeloid lineage cell types. These maturation abnormalities are known as myelodysplasia. In addition, blast cells may be found in the circulation (Figure 9.8). Cells with maturation abnormalities and blast cells can also be found in the peripheral blood of animals with acute myeloid leukemia. The differentiation between these two processes is due mainly to the number and type of ab-

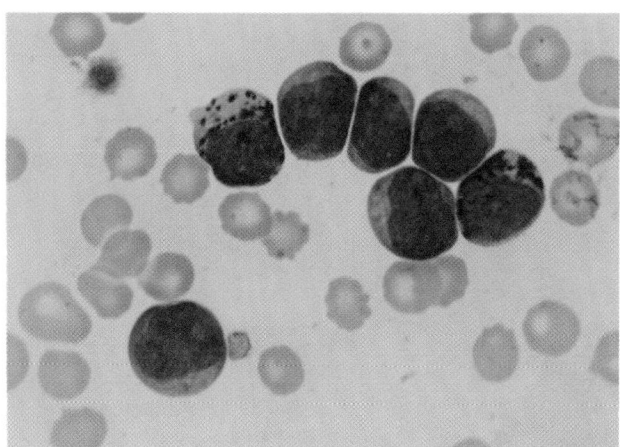

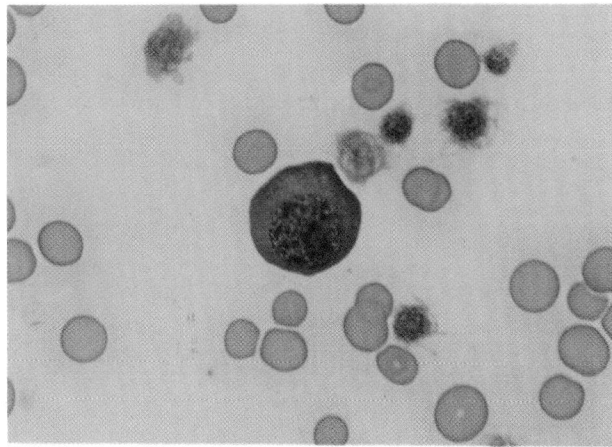

Figure 9.7. Large granular lymphocytic leukemia. This is a higher magnification of the blood smear shown in Figure 9.6. All the nucleated cells are large lymphocytes with often prominent nucleoli. Two of the cells have round to irregularly shaped, purple cytoplasmic granules. Canine blood smear, from 1989 ASVCP slide review, courtesy of M. Wellman; 100× objective.

Figure 9.8. Blast cell. Low numbers of blast cells may be found in the circulation of animals with myelodysplastic syndrome. The nucleated cell (center) with the round eccentrically placed nucleus, prominent single nucleolus, and moderate amounts of blue cytoplasm is a blast cell of probable erythrocytic origin. Giant platelets are present also. Feline blood smear; 100× objective.

normal cells present in the blood and bone marrow. Some myelodysplastic features found in the blood are described subsequently. Any given animal with myelodysplastic syndrome or myeloid leukemia may have one or more of these features.

Myelodysplasia of cells of the erythrocytic lineage is known as dyserythropoiesis. One feature of dyserythropoiesis is the formation of megaloblastic erythroid cells. These cells are recognized by their large size and dyssynchrony of maturation of the nucleus and cytoplasm. These cells often have mature-appearing reddish-orange cytoplasm, which is typical of red blood cells with their full hemoglobin content, and a large immature-appearing nucleus with noncondensed nuclear chromatin (Figure 9.9). Megaloblastosis also can be seen with B12 and folate deficiency, but this rarely has been documented in domestic animals.

A second feature of dyserythropoiesis is macrocytosis, which is characterized by high numbers of macrocytes, large red blood cells in circulation (Figure 9.10). Macrocytosis is commonly seen in regenerative anemias in all animals, but in myelodysplasia, macrocytosis typically occurs concurrently with a nonregenerative anemia. Macrocytic nonregenerative anemia also has been documented in a cat with folate deficiency. Macrocytosis occurs in some poodles and has little clinical significance. A third feature of dyserythropoiesis is the presence of sideroblasts and siderocytes, which, respectively, are nucleated or anucleated red blood cells with bluish granular material in the cytoplasm. This material is iron and can be difficult to distinguish from the common cause of basophilic stippling, which is RNA accumulation. A Prussian blue stain is necessary to confirm that the granular material is iron. Other abnormalities of erythrocytic differentiation that may be present include the presence of cells with multiple nuclei and abnormal nuclear shapes (Figure 9.11). Abnormal nuclear shapes of erythrocytic precursors have also been seen after the administration of vincristine.

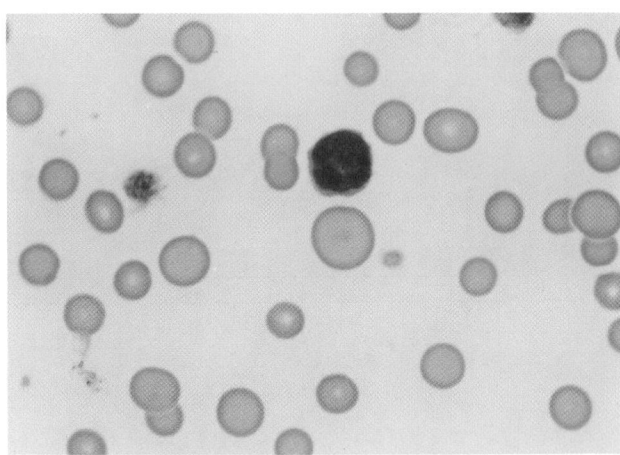

Figure 9.10. Macrocyte. The large, mature red blood cell in the center of the field directly below the lymphocyte is a macrocyte. Note the similarity of the size of this cell and the lymphocyte. If high numbers of macrocytes are present in an anemic animal with lack of polychromatophils, this is a feature of dyserythropoiesis. Feline blood smear; 100× objective.

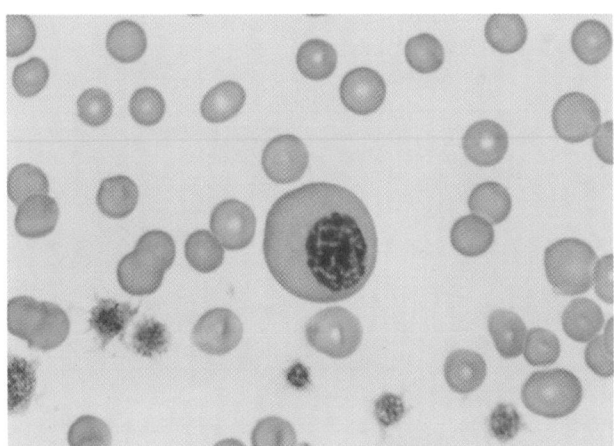

Figure 9.9. Megaloblastic, nucleated red blood cell. The large cell (center) with slightly eccentric, relatively immature, ovoid nucleus with condensed chromatin and bluish-red cytoplasm is a megaloblastic red blood cell precursor. The giant size and dyssynchrony in maturation of the cytoplasm and nucleus are features of dyserythropoiesis. Large platelets are also present. Feline blood smear; 100× objective.

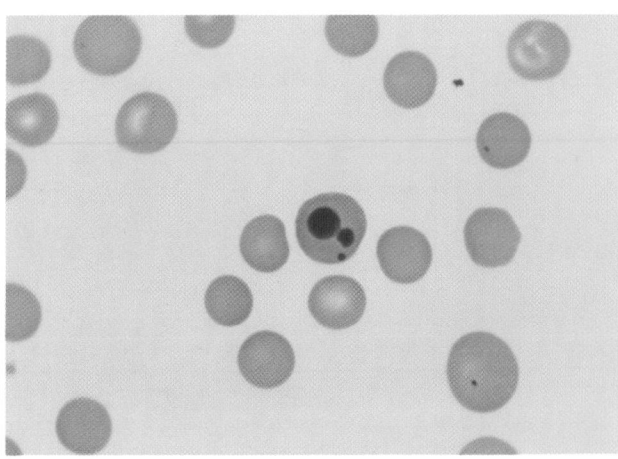

Figure 9.11. Abnormal nuclear shape. The metarubricyte in the center of the field has three variably sized, pyknotic nuclear fragments. This is a feature of dyserythropoiesis. Canine blood smear; 100× objective.

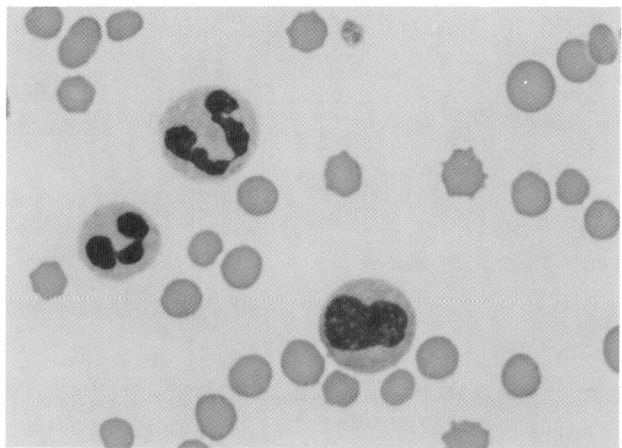

Figure 9.12. Giant neutrophil. The segmented neutrophil in the upper left corner is larger than the adjacent segmented neutrophil and metamyelocyte in the lower portion of the field. This may be a feature of dysgranulopoiesis. Feline blood smear; 100× objective.

Myelodysplasia of granulocytic development is known as dysgranulopoiesis. Nuclear changes that may be seen include hyper- and hyposegmentation as well as nuclear fragmentation. Changes in the cytoplasm of the cells include decreased numbers of granules or abnormal granule shapes, which can be most easily recognized in eosinophils or basophils. Giant neutrophils may be present also; however, enlarged neutrophils and possibly giant neutrophils may be seen as a sign of neutrophil toxicity during inflammatory disease (Figure 9.12).

Myelodysplasia of platelet production is known as dysthrombopoiesis. The main feature that may be present in the peripheral blood is a high number of giant platelets (Figures 9.13 and 9.14). These platelets may be hypo- or hypergranular. In cats, the presence of low to moderate numbers of giant platelets is common irrespective of the underlying disease state.

Acute Myeloid Leukemia

Acute Undifferentiated Leukemia The most poorly differentiated acute myeloid leukemia is acute undifferentiated leukemia. High numbers of cells that are very difficult to classify based on morphology as well as enzyme cytochemical staining patterns are present in the circulation. Included in this category is a disease in cats previously known as reticuloendotheliosis. In this disease, many blasts and immature-appearing cells are present in the circulation with some of the cells having eccentrically placed round nuclei with moderate amounts of blue cytoplasm with or without purple granules (Figure 9.15). The nuclear chromatin may be coarse and similar to cells of the erythrocytic lineage; however, cytoplasmic features are often similar to cells of the granulocytic lineage.

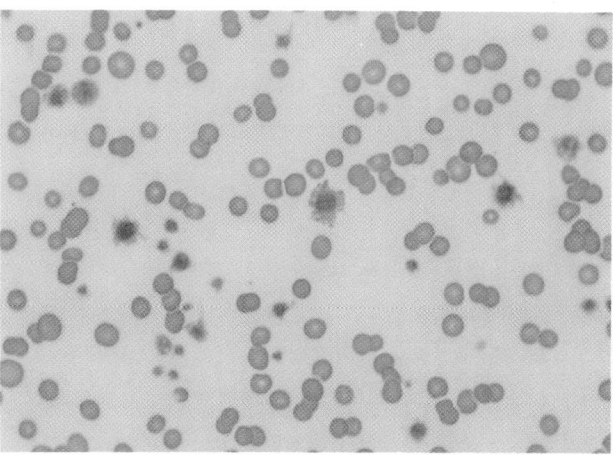

Figure 9.13. Giant platelets. Many giant platelets are present. Due to the high numbers and very large size of the platelets, this represents dysthrombopoiesis. Feline blood smear; 50× objective.

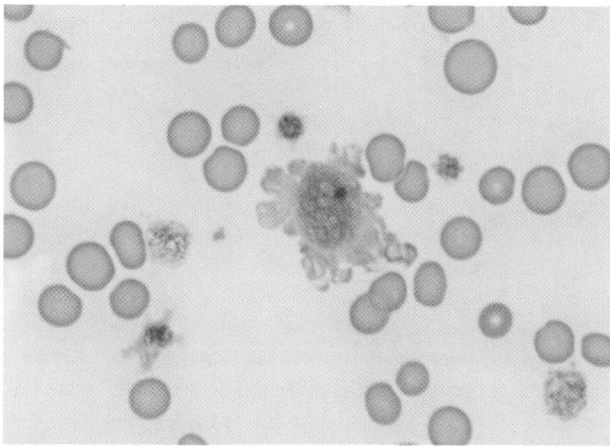

Figure 9.14. Giant platelet. This is a higher magnification of the blood smear shown in Figure 9.13. A very large, abnormally shaped giant platelet is present (center). Feline blood smear; 100× objective.

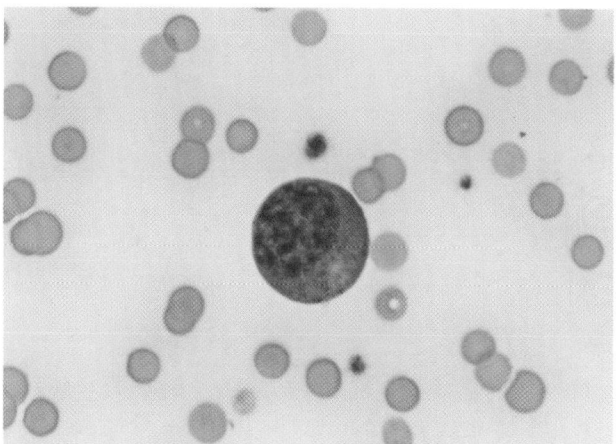

Figure 9.15. Acute undifferentiated leukemia. There is a very large cell (center) with a round to oval, eccentrically placed nucleus; a coarsely granular chromatin pattern; and moderate amounts of deep blue cytoplasm with pink-purple granules. This cell has features of both erythrocytic and granulocytic precursors. Feline blood smear; 100× objective.

Acute Myeloblastic Leukemia Acute myeloblastic leukemia, also known as acute granulocytic leukemia, has high numbers of immature granulocytic precursors in the peripheral blood. Typically, myeloblasts and possibly promyelocytes are present in high numbers (Figures 9.16 and 9.17). Other more mature granulocytic cells may be present; however, in contrast to severe inflammatory disease, these more mature granulocytes are in the minority. If just myeloblasts are present, it can be difficult to distinguish these cells from other blast cells such as lymphoblasts or monoblasts. In these cases, enzyme cytochemical staining is essential for accurate classification.

Acute Monocytic Leukemia Acute monocytic leukemia is recognized by the high number of monocytes as well as monocytic precursors, including promonocytes and monoblasts, in the circulation (Figures 9.18 and 9.19). Leukemias that just have monoblasts present can be difficult to distinguish from acute myeloblastic leukemia or acute lymphocytic leukemia.

Myelomonocytic Leukemia Myelomonocytic leukemia is a neoplastic proliferation of both types of cells of the granulocytic and monocytic lineage. It has the combined features of both acute myeloblastic leukemia and acute monocytic leukemia.

Erythroleukemia Erythroleukemia, as the name implies, is a leukemia of both red and white cell lineages. Both erythrocytic and leukocytic precursors are present in the circulation (Figures 9.20 and 9.21). An abnormal number of early precursors are typically present. This condition must be distinguished from a leukoerythroblastic state, which is a nonneoplastic process that occurs in times of extreme peripheral demand for red and white cells. The main way to distinguish these two when evaluating the blood smear is that, in erythroleukemia, there are typically a dispro-

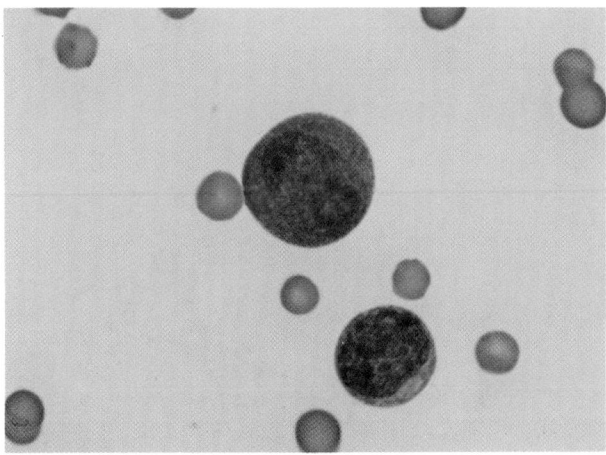

Figure 9.16. Acute myeloblastic (or acute granulocytic) leukemia. Four very large cells are present with round to indented, immature-appearing nuclei. Without cytochemical stains, these cells of the granulocytic lineage are difficult to distinguish from immature cells of the lymphocytic or monocytic lineage. Feline blood smear, from 1985 ASVCP slide review, courtesy of J. T. Blue; 100× objective.

Figure 9.17. Acute myeloblastic leukemia. Another field of view of the blood smear shown in Figure 9.16. The large cell in the center has an oval immature nucleus and pink cytoplasmic granules. The presence of the cytoplasmic granules similar to those of a normal promyelocyte help to classify this leukemia as granulocytic in origin. The smaller cell in the lower right may be a component of the leukemic process. Feline blood smear, from 1985 ASVCP slide review, courtesy of J. T. Blue; 100× objective.

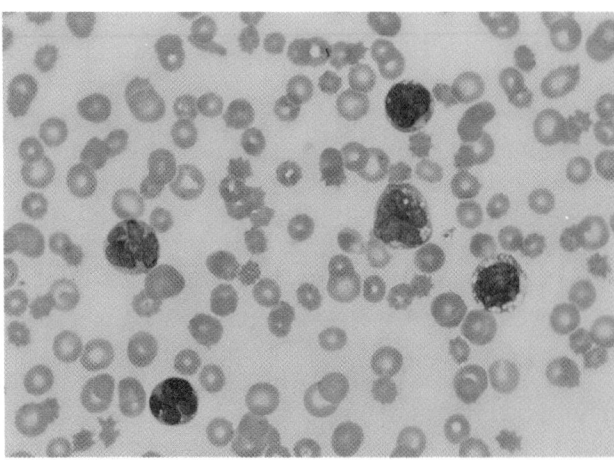

Figure 9.18. Acute monocytic leukemia. The five cells with deeply indented nuclei and occasionally vacuolated cytoplasm have features similar to normal monocytes. Canine blood smear; 50× objective.

portionate number of early erythrocytic and leukocytic precursors as compared with the number of mature cells. In contrast, during a leukoerythroblastic response, there are typically more mature erythrocytic and leukocytic precursors present than there are immature cells.

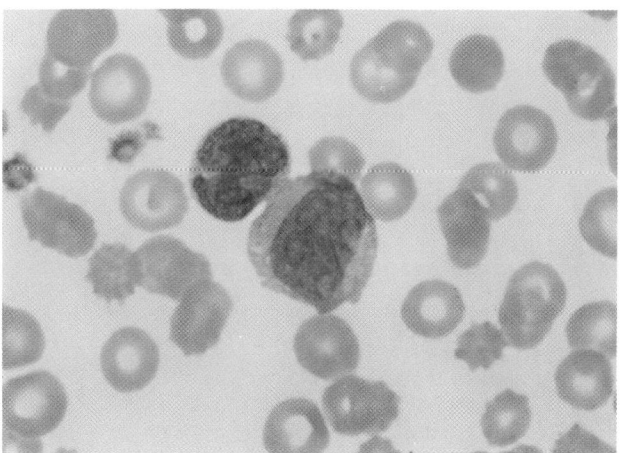

Figure 9.19. Acute monocytic leukemia. Another field of view of the blood smear shown in Figure 9.18. The large cell (center) with an oval nucleus and multiple, poorly distinct nucleoli is a monoblast. Due to the presence of high numbers of cells with monocytic morphology as shown in Figure 9.18 and monoblasts, this represents acute monocytic leukemia. Cytochemical staining for confirmation of cell lineage is recommended. Canine blood smear; 100× objective.

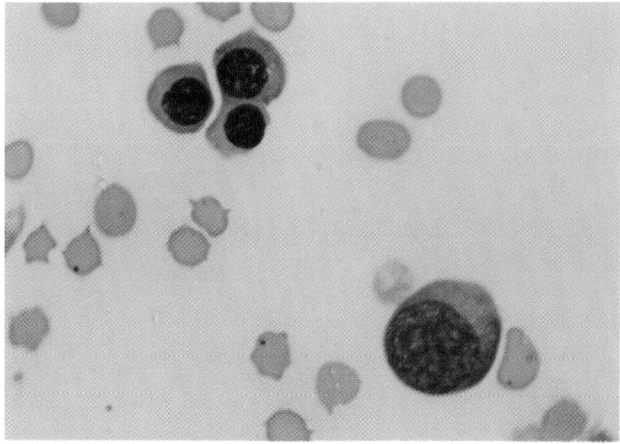

Figure 9.20. Erythroleukemia. Three nucleated red blood cells are present in the upper left corner. A large immature cell, probably an early granulocytic precursor, is present in the lower right corner. Feline blood smear; 100× objective.

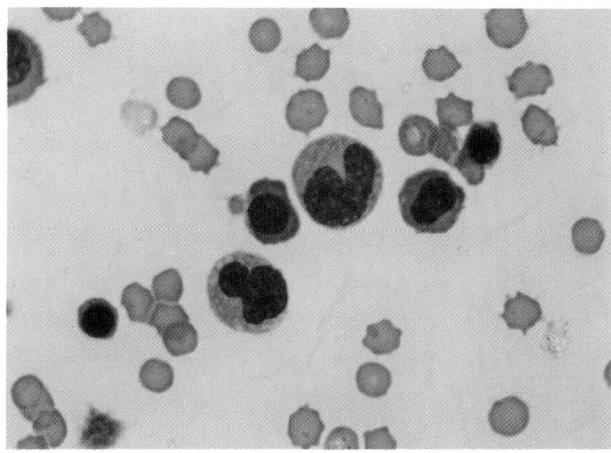

Figure 9.21. Erythroleukemia. Another field of view of the blood smear shown in Figure 9.20. Cells of the erythrocytic and granulocytic lineage are present. The presence of immature cells of the granulocytic and erythrocytic lineage, the decreased red blood cell density (anemia), and the lack of polychromatophils and mature, segmented neutrophils are representative of erythroleukemia. Feline blood smear; 100× objective.

Megakaryoblastic Leukemia Megakaryoblastic leukemia is recognized by the high number of megakaryoblasts in the circulation. As with other poorly differentiated leukemias, the megakaryoblasts may be difficult to differentiate from other blast cells based on morphology alone. Increases and decreases in platelet numbers as well as the presence of giant platelets and hypo- and hypergranulation of the platelets have also been documented.

Chronic Myeloid Leukemia

Chronic myeloid leukemia is recognized by high numbers of well-differentiated cells of the granulocytic lineage (neutrophilic, eosinophilic, or basophilic). These disorders are named by the predominant cell type present in the blood. For example, if mainly eosinophils are present, it is an eosinophilic leukemia. In these cases as well as other chronic myeloid leukemias, in addition to the presence of mature cells, immature cells may also be present. This can be seen in eosinophilic leukemia, whereby eosinophilic bands, metamyelocytes, and myelocytes may be present; however, the mature cell type vastly predominates. If cells of the neutrophilic lineage predominate, the disorder is known as chronic granulocytic or myelocytic leukemia (Figures 9.22 and 9.23).

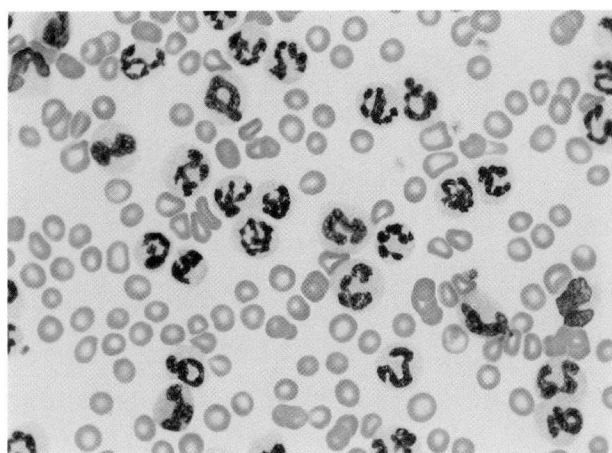

Figure 9.22. Chronic granulocytic leukemia. Many segmented neutrophils are present. The high numbers of neutrophils with a lack of inflammation present in this animal are diagnostic of chronic granulocytic leukemia. Canine blood smear; 50× objective.

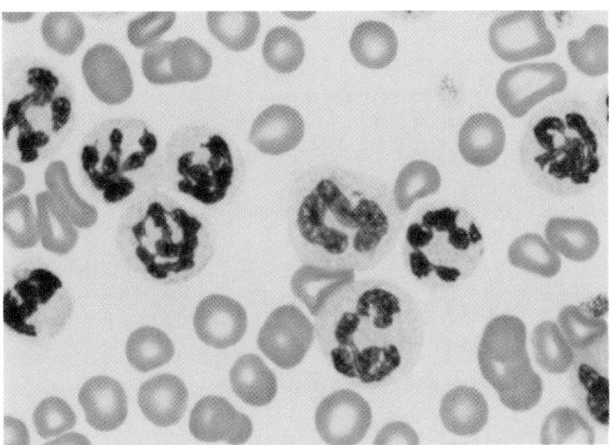

Figure 9.23. Chronic granulocytic leukemia. This is a higher magnification of the blood smear shown in Figure 9.22. Note the many segmented neutrophils present, the majority of which are hypersegmented. Canine blood smear; 100× objective.

Others

Erythremic Myelosis Erythremic myelosis has historically been classified as a leukemia of the erythrocytic lineage. This disorder has recently been renamed as either myelodysplastic syndrome with erythroid predominance or erythroleukemia with erythroid predominance, and mainly occurs in cats. In this disorder, erythrocytic precursors are present in the blood with a lack of significant numbers of polychromatophils (Figure 9.24). Most of the cells are usually metarubricytes and rubricytes, but prorubricytes and rubriblasts may be present also.

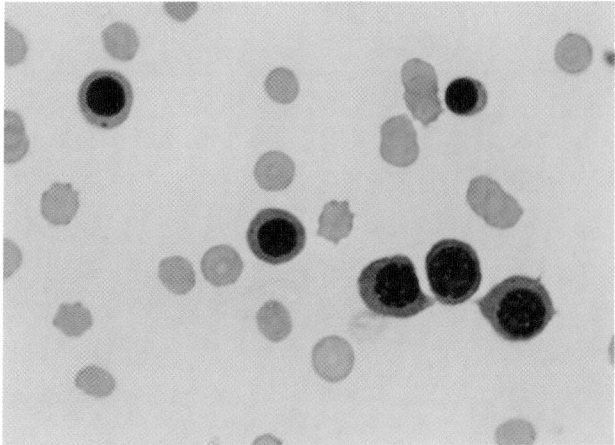

Figure 9.24. Erythremic myelosis. Six nucleated red blood cells are present. This finding associated with low red cell density (anemia) and a lack of polychromasia is supportive of erythremic myelosis. Feline blood smear; 100× objective.

Polycythemia Vera A well-differentiated leukemia of the erythrocytic lineage is known as polycythemia vera, in which there generally is not unusual morphology of the red blood cells; they are just present in very high numbers. Rarely, there have been reports of increased numbers of white blood cells in these animals as well. These findings suggest a multiple cell lineage affect, rather than a sole erythrocytic abnormality.

Essential Thrombocythemia A well-differentiated leukemia of the megakaryocytic lineage is known as essential thrombocythemia (Figure 9.25). Abnormal platelet morphology such as giant platelets and hypo- and hypergranulation of the platelets have been documented in addition to the marked thrombocytosis that is seen.

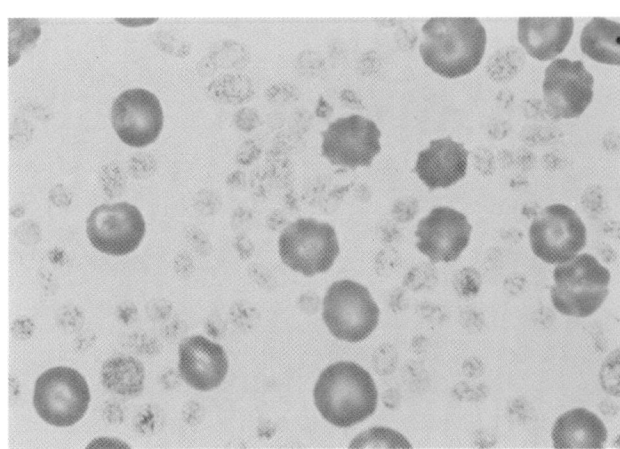

Figure 9.25. Marked thrombocytosis. Many platelets are present throughout the field. This extreme thrombocytosis is typical of essential thrombocythemia. Canine blood smear, from 1987 ASVCP slide review, courtesy of J. G. Zinkl; 100× objective.

Neoplastic Proliferation of Mast Cells Although not a true leukemia, neoplastic proliferation of mast cells may occur in the bone marrow with subsequent release of these cells into circulation (Figures 9.26 and 9.27). This can result in often finding high numbers of poorly to well-granulated mast cells in the circulation. Mast cells present in the circulation (mastocytemia) secondary to a neoplastic proliferation must be differentiated from mast cells in the circulation in association with inflammatory disease. Typically, when mast cells are found in the circulation secondary to inflammatory disease, the cells are well granulated and present in very low numbers. This, also, often is a very transient response.

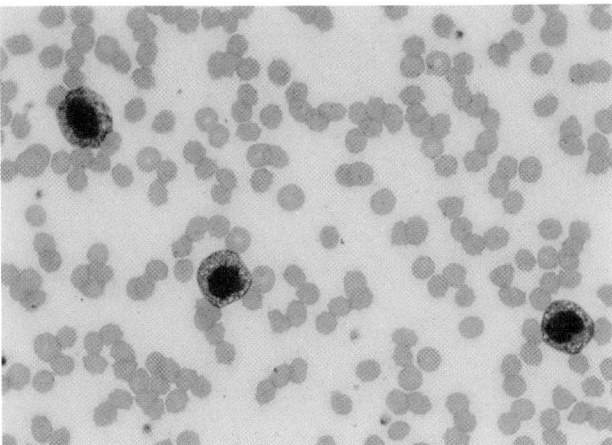

Figure 9.26. Mastocytemia. Three mast cells are present. If there is a high number of mast cells present in the circulation and inflammatory disease is not present, a systemic mast cell neoplastic process is likely. Feline blood smear; 50× objective.

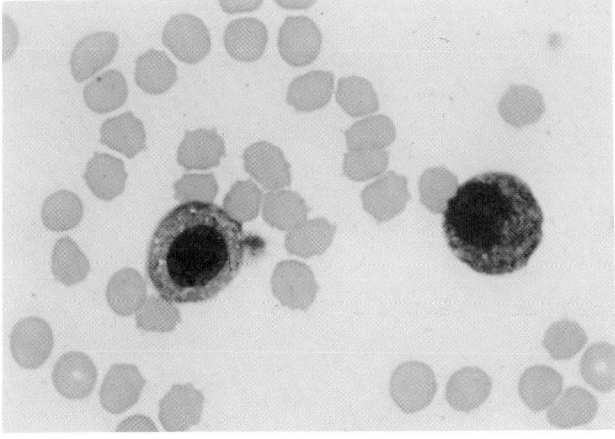

Figure 9.27. Mastocytemia. Another field from the blood smear shown in Figure 9.26. Two well-granulated mast cells are present. Feline blood smear; 100× objective.

CHAPTER TEN

MISCELLANEOUS FINDINGS

There are several different cell types that are often not classified accurately by the novice. These cell types are contrasted here. Small lymphocytes are sometimes confused with nucleated red blood cells, specifically rubricytes (Figure 10.1). Both of these cells have very high nuclear to cytoplasmic ratios and round nuclei. The main difference is the chromatin pattern of the nuclei. Small lymphocytes have a homogeneous, glassy- to smudged-appearing nuclear chromatin with some areas of condensation. In contrast, rubricytes have a much more coarsely granular and clumped nuclear chromatin. The color of the cytoplasm may also be helpful. The cytoplasm of the rubricyte ranges from deep blue to reddish-blue, whereas the cytoplasm of the small lymphocyte is typically light blue but may be deep blue if reactive.

Large lymphocytes are sometimes confused with monocytes, which do not have vacuoles in the cytoplasm (Figure 10.2). Both cells have a moderate nuclear to cytoplasmic ratio. Large lymphocyte nuclei are typically round to oval but may be indented. In contrast, monocyte nuclei may be round to oval but usually have multiple indentations. The chromatin pattern of the large lymphocyte is more homogeneous

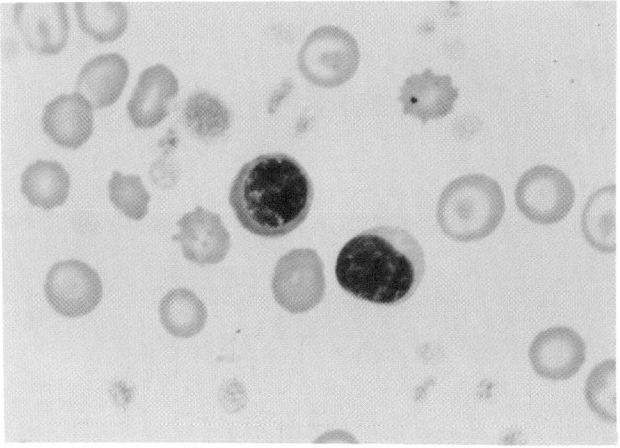

Figure 10.1. Rubricyte versus lymphocyte. The cell (left of center) with a round nucleus with very clumped chromatin and rim of reddish-blue cytoplasm is a rubricyte. The cell (right of center) with a round to oval, slightly indented nucleus and smudged nuclear chromatin with some areas of condensation is a small lymphocyte. Note that the cytoplasm of the lymphocyte is light blue compared with the reddish-blue cytoplasm of the rubricyte. Canine blood smear; 100× objective.

compared with the net-like chromatin with several clumped areas of the monocyte. Both cells have blue cytoplasm; however, the cytoplasm of the monocyte is typically more blue-gray. If a large cell that may be a monocyte or lymphocyte is observed, it may be useful to find a more classic monocyte with vacuoles and compare this cell with the cell in question and see if the nuclear chromatin and color of the cytoplasm are similar or different.

Monocytes also are sometimes confused with toxic band neutrophils and metamyelocytes. Differentiating these cells is one of the great challenges in cell identification (Figure 10.3). Monocytes, toxic band neutrophils, and metamyelocytes are often of similar size with blue cytoplasm. The nucleus of the monocyte can be band- or kidney bean-shaped, similar to the nucleus of the band neutrophil and metamyelocyte, respectively. One of the primary differences among these three cell types is related to the nuclear chromatin patterns. The monocyte nuclear chromatin is lacy or net-like with some areas of condensation, and the chromatin of the cells of the neutrophilic lineage is more condensed or clumped. The presence of Döhle bodies is helpful in accurately identifying the cell as an immature neutrophil also; Döhle bodies are not present in monocytes.

Other miscellaneous cell types include smudge, pyknotic, and mitotic cells. Smudge cells are just broken cells (Figure 10.4), and it is impossible to accurately identify their exact origin. Typically, however, they will not have intact cell membranes and the cytoplasm is lost; only free nuclear chromatin material is present. These cells are sometimes also called basket cells, because of the delicate, woven basket-like strands of dispersed nuclear chromatin. Low numbers of these cells may be present in normal preparations. High numbers of broken cells may be present if the blood sample is lipemic or, sometimes, when high numbers of neoplastic and possibly more-fragile cells are present.

Cells that are undergoing pyknosis, which is a natural process of cell injury and death, have very condensed nuclear chromatin (Figure 10.5). It is often impossible to tell the origin of pyknotic cells. The pyknotic nuclear bodies may undergo fragmentation, and many small pieces of condensed nuclear material may be present.

Mitotic cells are cells that are dividing and thus the

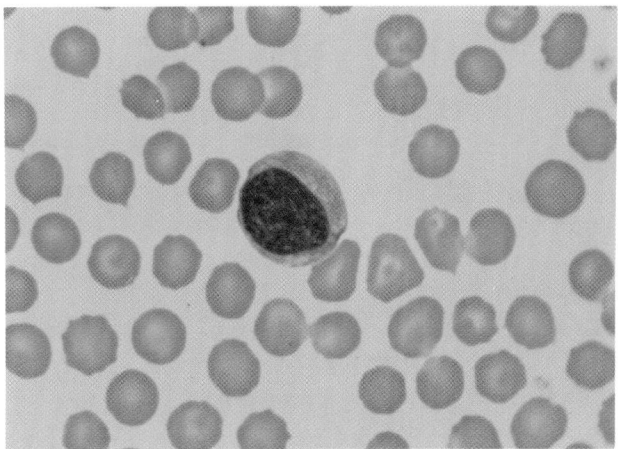

Figure 10.2. Large lymphocyte. The cell with the oval nucleus and moderate amount of light blue cytoplasm is a large lymphocyte. Note the chromatin is more homogeneous compared with the net-like chromatin with areas of condensation of the monocytes in Figure 10.3. Canine blood smear; 100× objective.

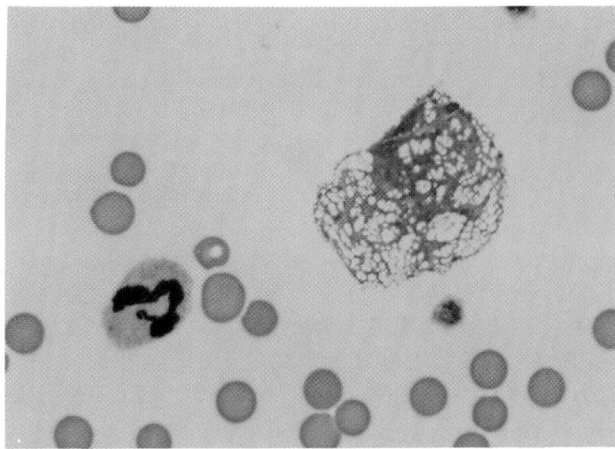

Figure 10.4. Smudge cell. The large, light purple, net-like structure in the right center of the field is a broken, or smudge, cell; this is free nuclear chromatin material. There is a neutrophil present (lower left). Feline blood smear; 100× objective.

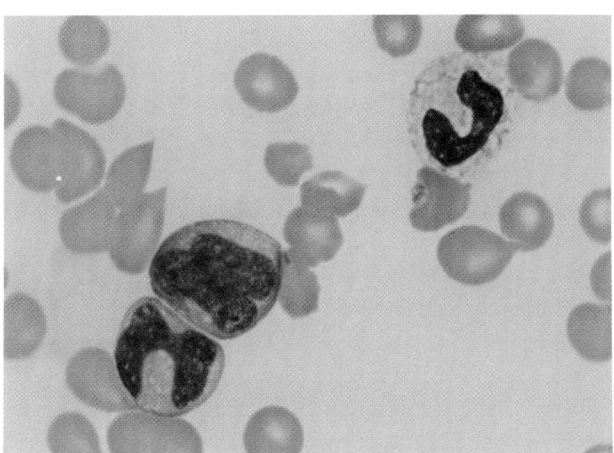

Figure 10.3. Monocyte versus toxic band neutrophil. The two nucleated cells in the lower left quadrant are monocytes; the large nucleated cell in the upper right quadrant is a toxic band neutrophil. Note that the chromatin pattern of the band neutrophil is much more condensed or clumped compared with the more open, net-like chromatin pattern of the monocyte. Canine blood smear; 100× objective.

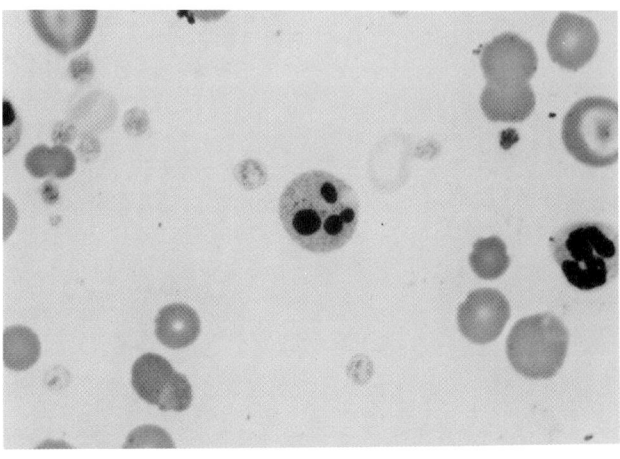

Figure 10.5. Pyknotic cell. The cell (center) with pink cytoplasm and four markedly condensed nuclear fragments is a pyknotic neutrophil. There is a normal segmented neutrophil present to the right of the pyknotic neutrophil. Canine blood smear; 100× objective.

chromosomes are visible (Figure 10.6). The exact origin of the mitotic cells is often impossible to identify. It is uncommon to see these in the peripheral blood, but if they are present in significant numbers, a neoplastic process may be present.

Cell identification often depends on recognizing the color of the cell, which in turn depends on the type and quality of the stain used. A commonly used,

rapid, modified Wright's stain is Diff-Quik®. With this stain, the color of the blood cells is slightly different compared with the color of the cells in the photomicrographs shown throughout the text, which are Wright's stained. One of the major color differences is that of the red blood cells. Often, the mature red blood cells stain bluish-gray to brownish-red with Diff-Quik® (Figure 10.7). Polychromatophils may be diffi-

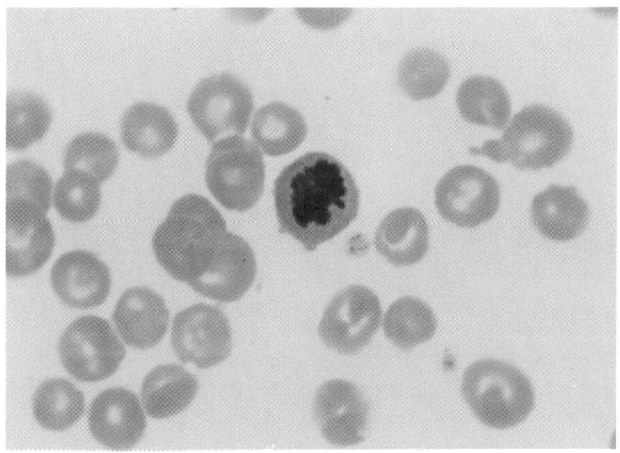

Figure 10.6. Mitotic figure. The blue cell with an irregularly shaped nucleus is a cell undergoing mitosis. Canine blood smear; 100× objective.

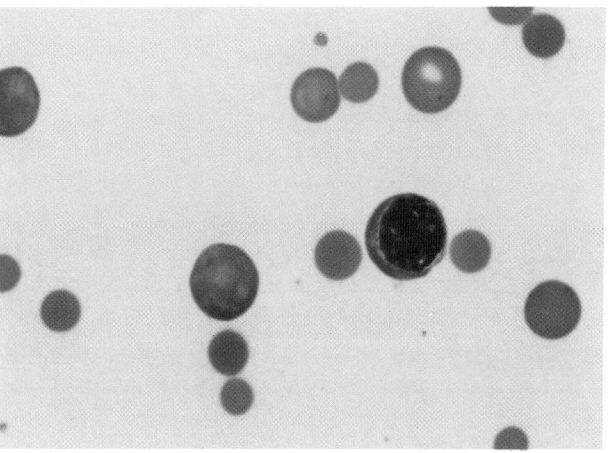

Figure 10.8. Rubricyte. The cell in the right center of the field is a rubricyte. Note the marked clumped chromatin compared with the rubricyte shown in Figure 10.1. Polychromatophils (larger and bluish-purple–staining cells) and mature red blood cells are present also. Bovine blood smear; Diff-Quik® stain; 100× objective.

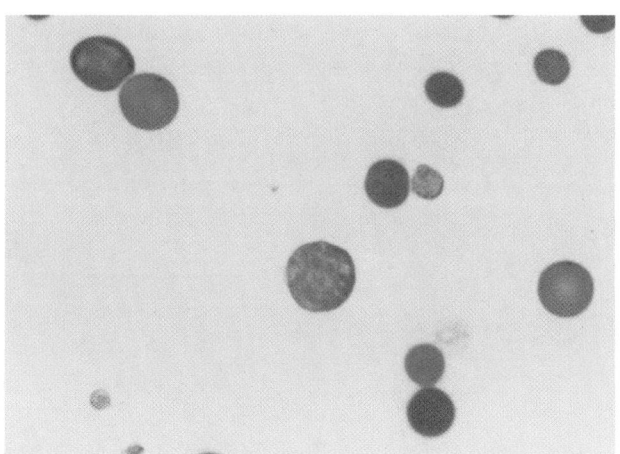

Figure 10.7. Mature red blood cells and polychromatophils. The bluish-purple cells in the center of the field and upper left corner are polychromatophils. The other cells are mature red blood cells and platelets. Bovine blood smear; Diff-Quik® stain; 100× objective.

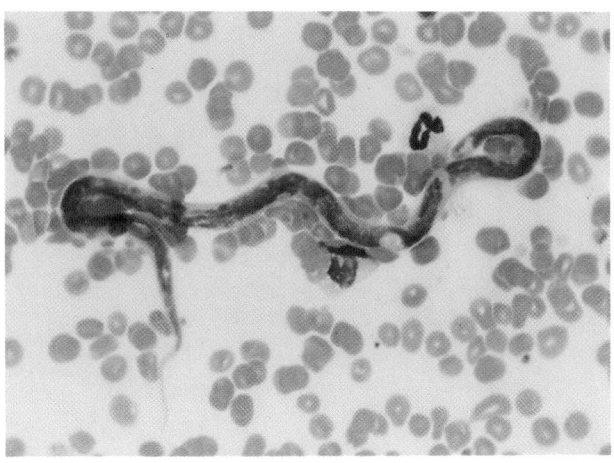

Figure 10.9. Microfilaria. The very large, elongated structure in the center of the field is a microfilaria. Canine blood smear; 50× objective.

cult to identify because they stain bluish-red to bluish-purple. The cytoplasm of the neutrophils, also, often is more blue, which may be confused with mild toxicity. Finally, the chromatin of most of the nucleated cells is often more accentuated or clumped when Diff-Quik® stain is used (Figure 10.8).

Two extracellular organisms that may be present in the blood are microfilaria and trypanosomes. Microfi-

laria are easily recognized, based on their very large size. Typically, they are a few hundred microns long and several microns thick (Figure 10.9). Due to their large size, the organisms often end up on the feathered edge of the blood smear. The two most commonly recognized microfilaria are *Dirofilaria immitis* and *Dipetalonema reconditum*, which are most often found in dogs. Several characteristics, including length, shape, and thickness, can be used to distinguish these two different types of microfilaria. These features are best evaluated in wet mounts or fixed preparations. Generally, if microfilaria are present on an air-dried blood smear, they are reported as just microfilaria and other tests are necessary for accurate classification. Trypanosomes are rarely seen in the peripheral blood of animals but their significance varies from area to area. Of the widely distributed nonpathogenic species, *Trypanosoma theileri* in cattle (Figure 10.10) in North America, Western Europe, and Australia and *T. melophagium* in sheep are the most common. Pathogenic trypanosomes are important parasites and may be found in horses and cattle in tropical and subtropical zones. *Trypanosoma cruzi* in dogs is mainly found in the United States and South and Central America. These are large, elongated, ribbon-like structures, often with tapered ends. They frequently have an indistinct, undulating membrane on one side and a small, round, deeply staining internal structure known as a kinetoplast. *T. theileri* are 25 to 120 μm long. *T. cruzi* are 16 to 20 μm long.

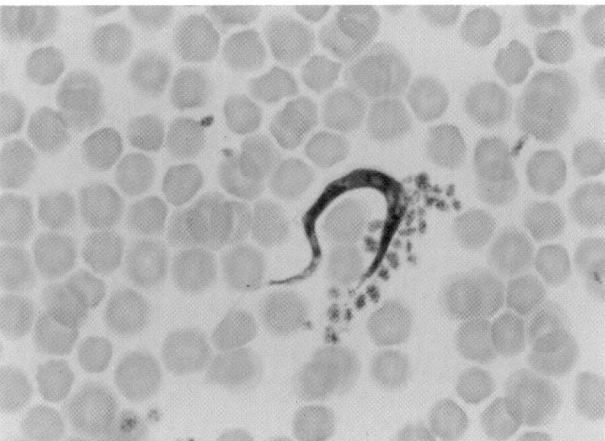

Figure 10.10. *Trypanosoma theileri.* The ribbon-like structure with tapered ends is typical of trypanosome species. This specimen is surrounded by a clump of platelets. Notice the faintly staining membrane along the convex border and the elongate, delicate flagellum at one end. Bovine blood smear; 100× objective.

Appendixes

Appendix 1: Semiquantitative Grading Scheme for Evaluation of Red Blood Cell Morphology*

Morphology and Species	Grading Scheme			
	1+	2+	3+	4+
Anisocytosis				
Dog	7–15	16–20	21–29	>30
Cat	5–8	9–15	16–20	>20
Cow	10–20	21–30	31–40	>40
Horse	1–3	4–6	7–10	>10
Polychromasia				
Dog	2–7	8–14	15–29	>30
Cat	1–2	3–8	9–15	>15
Cow	2–5	6–10	11–20	>20
Horse	. . . . rarely observed			
Hypochromasia				
All Species	1–10	11–50	51–200	>200
Poikilocytosis				
All Species	3–10	11–50	51–200	>200
Target Cells				
Dogs Only	3–5	6–15	16–30	>30
Spherocytes				
All Species	1–10	11–50	51–150	>150
Miscellaneous Morphology (Acanthocytes, Schistocytes, Dacryocytes, Heinz bodies, Howell-Jolly bodies, etc.)				
All Species	1–2	3–8	9–20	>20
Basophilic Stippling				
All Species	. . . . report as noted when observed			

Source: Adapted from Table 3 by Weiss, Douglass J. 1984. Uniform evaluation and semiquantitative reporting of hematologic data in veterinary laboratories. *Veterinary Clinical Pathology* 13(2):27-31. Permission granted by Veterinary Practice Publishing Company.

*Red blood cell morphology is assessed as the average number of abnormal cells in the monolayer of the smear using the 100x objective. When using this table, a monolayer is defined as a microscopic field in which approximately half of the red blood cells are touching each other.

APPENDIX 2: SEMIQUANTITATIVE GRADING SCHEME FOR EVALUATION OF NEUTROPHIL TOXICITY

Neutrophil toxicity*

  1+ Mild basophilia

  2+ Moderate basophilia and/or mild foamy cytoplasm and Döhle bodies may be noted

  3+ Marked basophilia and/or marked foamy cytoplasm and Döhle bodies may be noted

  4+ Criteria similar to 3+ with indistinct nuclear membranes

*In cats and horses, Döhle bodies may be present without other signs of toxicity; if so, the following classification would be used.

  1+ <10% of neutrophils contain Döhle bodies

  2+ 10 to 30% of neutrophils contain Döhle bodies

  3+ >30% of neutrophils contain Döhle bodies

Glossary

Acanthocyte   A red blood cell with multiple, variably sized, irregular membrane projections that are due to alterations in the ratio of membrane cholesterol to phospholipids.

Agglutination   Clumping of red blood cells that is usually due to cross-linking of red blood cell surface–associated antibodies.

Agranulocyte   A white blood cell that does not contain secondary granules. The two types of agranulocytes are lymphocytes and monocytes.

Anemia   A condition in which the hemoglobin, packed cell volume, and red blood cell count decrease below the normal reference range.

Anisocytosis   A variation in the size of cells; in hematology, this is most often used to describe variation in the size of red blood cells.

Azurophilic granules   Cytoplasmic granules that stain pink to reddish-purple with Wright's stain.

Band cell   A type of white blood cell with a nuclear membrane that has parallel sides, although slight indentations may be present. Band cells can be of the neutrophilic, eosinophilic, or basophilic lineage.

Bar cell   A red blood cell with a central bar-shaped outfolding. This cell is also known as a knizocyte.

Basophil   A white blood cell of the granulocytic lineage with a segmented nucleus, purple cytoplasm, and often purple cytoplasmic granules.

Basophilia   The reaction of a cell to Wright's stain resulting in a bluish-stained cytoplasm; also describes the color of the cytoplasm of toxic neutrophils or refers to an increase in the number of basophils in the circulation.

Basophilic   A bluish color on Wright's-stained preparations; also refers to basophils.

Basophilic stippling   The presence of very small, dark blue staining bodies within the red blood cell. The stippling is usually due to RNA accumulation but may be associated with iron accumulation.

Blister cell   A red blood cell with a membrane vacuole.

Bone marrow   The central portion of long, flat, and irregular bones that is the principle site of hematopoiesis.

Buffy coat   A layer of white blood cells and platelets that collects immediately above the red blood cells in centrifuged whole blood; it has a whitish appearance.

Burr cell   An oval to elongated red blood cell with multiple, fine projections.

Chromatin   A complex of DNA and nuclear proteins.

Codocyte   A red blood cell with an extra round outfolding of membrane in the middle of the cell that gives the cell a target-like appearance. This cell is commonly known as a target cell.

Crenation   An in vitro artifact that results in the formation of red blood cells with multiple, regular-shaped, small fine points on the cell membrane.

Cytoplasm   The portion of the cell that is exclusive of the nucleus.

Dacryocyte   A teardrop-shaped red blood cell that may be seen in animals with myelofibrosis.

Deoxyribonucleic acid (DNA) The nucleic acid that contains the basic genetic information found in the nuclei of cells.

Diff-Quik® A commercially available preparation for manually staining slides with a modified Wright's stain.

Disseminated intravascular coagulation (DIC) A pathophysiological state that may develop due to damage of endothelial cells, activation of platelets, and activation of the coagulation system. This results in often severe life-threatening bleeding abnormalities.

Döhle body A small, round to irregular, blue structure in the cytoplasm of cells of the neutrophilic lineage. It is an abnormal aggregate of RNA in the cell and one sign of toxicity.

Dyserythropoiesis Myelodysplasia of cells of the erythrocytic lineage.

Dysgranulopoiesis Myelodysplasia of cells of the granulocytic lineage.

Dysthrombopoiesis Myelodysplasia of platelets.

Eccentrocyte A red blood cell with a crescent-shaped clear area that is eccentrically placed. This cell is formed due to oxidant-induced damage to the red blood cell membranes.

Echinocyte A red blood cell with multiple, small, delicate, regular-shaped spines distributed evenly around the membrane. The most common cause of echinocyte formation is an in vitro artifact known as crenation.

Eosinophil A white blood cell of the granulocytic lineage with reddish to reddish-orange granules in the cytoplasm.

Erythrocyte A mature red blood cell.

Erythropoiesis The production of red blood cells.

Ethylenediaminetetraacetate (EDTA) The anticoagulant most commonly used for the collection of blood for hematological examination.

Ghost cell A remnant membrane of a red blood cell.

Granulocyte A white blood cell that contains secondary, also known as specific, cytoplasmic granules. The three different types of granulocytes are neutrophils, eosinophils, and basophils.

Granulopoiesis The production of granulocytes, which include cells of the neutrophilic, basophilic, and eosinophilic lineages.

Heinz body A rounded, often refractile, projection from the surface of the red blood cell that is due to oxidation and denaturation of hemoglobin.

Hematocrit The percentage of red blood cells relative to plasma.

Hematology The study of blood.

Hematopoiesis The production of blood cells.

Hemoglobin The protein in red blood cells that carries oxygen.

Hemosiderin The insoluble form of iron that appears as golden-brown to black, granular to globular material.

Howell-Jolly body A small piece of remnant nuclear material in the red blood cell.

Hypochromasia The presence of red blood cells in the circulation that have increased central pallor and decreased staining intensity of the membrane due to decreased hemoglobin content.

Hypochromic cell A red blood cell with increased central pallor and decreased staining intensity of the membrane.

Keratocyte A red blood cell with two fairly uniform horn-like projections.

Knizocyte A red blood cell with a central bar-shaped outfolding. This cell is also known as a bar cell.

Left shift An increase in the number of band neutrophils and other immature cells of the granulocytic lineage in the peripheral blood.

Leptocyte A red blood cell, which, typically, is larger with excessive, thin membranes and folds easily. Target cells and bar cells are types of leptocytes.

Leukemia A neoplastic proliferation of cells of bone marrow origin that are usually released into the blood.

Leukemoid Pertaining to the presence of very high numbers of neutrophilic granulocytes in the circulation, often with many immature forms; due to the degree of elevation of the white blood cell count, this may be confused with a true leukemia.

Leukocyte A white blood cell.

Lymphocyte A white blood cell of the agranulocytic lineage that is characterized by a round nucleus and light blue cytoplasm. There are two main types: B lymphocytes, which develop into plasma cells and produce antibodies, and T lymphocytes, which are important in the cellular immune response.

Lymphoproliferative disorder A clonal neoplastic proliferation of cells of the lymphocytic lineage.

Macrocyte A red blood cell that is larger than normal.

Macrophage A large phagocytic cell found in tissues such as the bone marrow; this cell develops from a blood monocyte.

Mast cell A granulated round cell found in low numbers in the bone marrow.

Medullary Pertaining to bone marrow.

Megakaryocyte A very large cell that produces platelets and is found in the bone marrow.

Metamyelocyte The stage of development of granulocytes between the myelocyte and the band cell.

Metarubricyte The stage of development of red blood cells between the rubricyte and the polychromatophil.

Mitotic cell A cell that is undergoing division; the chromosomes are visible.

Monocyte A white blood cell of the agranulocytic lineage that is characterized by a variably shaped nucleus and blue-gray cytoplasm, which is frequently vacuolated.

Myeloblast The cell that is the earliest microscopically identifiable stage of development of granulocytes found in the bone marrow.

Myelocyte The stage of development of granulocytes between the promyelocyte and the metamyelocyte.

Myelodysplasia Alterations in the normal development and maturation of cells of the myeloid lineage.

Myelofibrosis A condition in which the bone marrow has varying degrees of increased fibrous connective tissue that displaces the normal blood cell precursors.

Myeloid Pertaining to the bone marrow. More specifically, this term is used to collectively describe the cells of the granulocytic, erythrocytic, megakaryocytic, and monocytic lineages.

Myeloproliferative disorder A clonal neoplastic proliferation of cells of the myeloid lineage.

Neutrophil A white blood cell of the granulocytic lineage with a segmented nucleus and pink to light blue cytoplasm.

New methylene blue stain A stain used to identify reticulocytes and to more readily see Heinz bodies.

Nonregenerative anemia An anemia in which there is not adequate production of red blood cells in the bone marrow.

Nucleolus A small round structure in the nuclei of cells that contains RNA and protein; it usually stains bluish with Wright's stain. Nucleoli (pl.).

Nucleus The central spherical structure within a cell that contains DNA, nucleoli, and nuclear proteins. Nuclei (pl.).

Osteoblast A cell in the bone marrow, found in low numbers, that is important in bone formation.

Osteoclast   A very large multinucleated cell in the bone marrow that is important in bone remodeling.

Ovalocyte   An oval-shaped red blood cell.

Packed cell volume (PCV)   The percentage of red blood cells relative to plasma, determined by centrifugation.

Pappenheimer bodies   Iron inclusions in red blood cells that appear as pale blue granules with Wright's stain.

Plasma   The fluid noncellular portion of anticoagulated whole blood.

Plasma cell   An oval cell with eccentric nuclei; it may be found in the bone marrow and produces antibody.

Platelet   A small, anucleated cytoplasmic fragment from megakaryocytes that is present in the peripheral blood and is important in hemostasis. This cell is also known as a thrombocyte.

Poikilocytosis   The presence of abnormally shaped red blood cells in the circulation.

Polychromasia   The presence of polychromatophils in the blood.

Polychromatophil   An immature red blood cell that is typically larger than the mature red blood cell and stains bluish to bluish-red with Wright's stain.

Promyelocyte   The stage of development of granulocytes between the myeloblast and the myelocyte.

Prorubricyte   The stage of development of red blood cells between the rubriblast and the rubricyte.

Punched-out cell   A red blood cell with accentuated central pallor. This cell is also known as a torocyte.

Pyknotic cell   A cell with a small nucleus and very condensed chromatin.

Reactive lymphocyte   A lymphocyte with a dark blue cytoplasm and, sometimes, a perinuclear clear zone. Also, the cell may be larger than a typical small lymphocyte.

Red blood cell (RBC)   An anucleated cell that stains reddish to reddish-orange with Wright's stain. The main function of the red blood cell is to carry oxygen.

Regenerative anemia   An anemia in which there is an increase in production of red blood cells in the bone marrow, with subsequent release into the peripheral blood.

Reticular   Resembling a net.

Reticulocyte   An immature erythrocyte that contains clumps of ribosomal RNA and mitochondria, which stain with new methylene blue. These cells correspond to polychromatophils seen in Wright's-stained preparations.

Ribonucleic acid (RNA)   The nucleic acid that is important in protein synthesis.

Rough endoplasmic reticulum   A cytoplasmic organelle that is important in protein synthesis.

Rouleaux   Organized linear arrays and sometimes branching chains of red blood cells.

Rubriblast   The cell that is the earliest microscopically identifiable stage of development of red blood cells found in the bone marrow.

Rubricyte   A stage of development of red blood cells between the prorubricyte and the metarubricyte.

Schistocyte   An irregularly shaped fragment of a red blood cell.

Sideroblast   A nucleated red blood cell that contains Pappenheimer bodies.

Siderocyte   An anucleated red blood cell that contains Pappenheimer bodies.

Smudge cell   A cell with no intact cell membrane but only free nuclear chromatin material. This cell is sometimes called a basket cell because of the delicate, woven, basket-like strands of dispersed nuclear chromatin.

Spherocyte   A smaller-appearing red blood cell that lacks central pallor and is usually a result of immune-mediated damage to the cell.

Stomatocyte A red blood cell with central pallor that is oval to elongated and takes on the appearance of a mouth.

Target cell A red blood cell with an extra round outfolding of membrane in the middle of the cell that gives the cell a target-like appearance. This cell is also known as a codocyte.

Thrombocyte A small, anucleated cytoplasmic fragment from a megakaryocyte that is present in the peripheral blood and important in hemostasis. This cell is also known as a platelet.

Torocyte A red blood cell with accentuated central pallor. This cell is commonly known as a punched-out cell.

Toxicity A group of morphological changes during inflammation that may be present in cells of the neutrophilic lineage. The three main features of toxicity are increased basophilia, foaminess, and the presence of Döhle bodies in the cytoplasm.

White blood cell (WBC) A nucleated cell in the blood that does not contain hemoglobin. This cell is also known as a leukocyte. The two major types of white blood cells are granulocytes and agranulocytes.

Selected References

Alleman, A.R., and Harvey, J.W. 1993. The morphologic effects of vincristine sulfate on canine bone marrow cells. Veterinary Clinical Pathology 22(2): 36–41.

Duncan, J. Robert; Prasse, Keith W.; and Mahaffey, Edward A. 1994. Veterinary Laboratory Medicine: Clinical Pathology, 3rd ed. Ames: Iowa State University Press.

Fox, J.C.; Ewing, S.A.; Buckner, R.G.; Whitenack, D.; and Manley, J.H. 1986. *Trypanosoma cruzi* infection in a dog from Oklahoma. Journal of the American Veterinary Medical Association 189(12): 1583–1584.

Fyfe, John C.; Jezyk, Peter F.; Giger, Urs; and Patterson, Donald F. 1989. Inherited selective malabsorption of vitamin B12 in giant schnauzers. Journal of the American Animal Hospital Association 25: 533–539.

Glenn, Bertis L., and Stair, Ernest L. 1984. Cytauxzoonosis in domestic cats: Report of two cases in Oklahoma, with a review and discussion of the disease. Journal of the American Veterinary Medical Association 184(7): 822–825.

Jain, Nemi C. 1986. Schalms Veterinary Hematology, 4th ed. Philadelphia: Lea and Febiger.

Jain, Nemi C. 1993. Essentials of Veterinary Hematology. Philadelphia: Lea and Febiger.

Latimer, Kenneth S. 1995. Leukocytes in health and disease. In Textbook of Veterinary Internal Medicine: Diseases of the Dog and Cat, 4th ed., vol. 2, pp. 1892–1929. Ed. Stephen J. Ettinger and Edward C. Feldman. Philadelphia: W.B. Saunders Company.

Myers, S.; Wiks, K.; and Giger, U. 1995. Macrocytic anemia caused by naturally-occurring folate-deficiency in the cat. Veterinary Pathology 32(5): 547.

Reagan, William J., and Rebar, Alan H. 1995. Platelet disorders. In Textbook of Veterinary Internal Medicine: Diseases of the Dog and Cat, 4th ed., vol. 2, pp. 1964–1976. Ed. Stephen J. Ettinger and Edward C. Feldman. Philadelphia: W.B. Saunders Company.

Reagan, W.J.; Garry, F.; Thrall, M.A.; Colgan, S.; Hutchison, J.; and Weiser, M.G. 1990. The clinicopathologic, light, and scanning electron microscopic features of eperythrozoonosis in four naturally infected llamas. Veterinary Pathology 27: 426–431.

Rich, Lon J. 1976. The Morphology of Canine and Feline Blood Cells. Missouri: Ralston Purina Company.

Taboada, Joseph, and Merchant, Sandra R. 1995. Protozoal and miscellaneous infections. In Textbook of Veterinary Internal Medicine: Diseases of the Dog and Cat, 4th ed., vol. 1, pp. 384–397. Ed. Stephen J. Ettinger and Edward C. Feldman. Philadelphia: W.B. Saunders Company.

Van Houten, D.; Weiser, M.G.; Johnson, L.; and Garry, F. 1992. Reference hematologic values and morphologic features of blood cells in healthy adult llamas. American Journal of Veterinary Research 53(10): 1773–1779.

Weiser, M.G. 1995. Erythrocyte responses and disorders. In Textbook of Veterinary Internal Medicine: Diseases of the Dog and Cat, 4th ed., vol. 2, pp. 1864–1891. Ed. Stephen J. Ettinger and Edward C. Feldman. Philadelphia: W.B. Saunders Company.

Weiss, Douglas J. 1984. Uniform evaluation and semiquantitative reporting of hematologic data in veterinary laboratories. Veterinary Clinical Pathology 13(2): 27–31.

Williard, Michael D.; Tvedten, Harold; and Turnwald, Grant H. 1989. Small Animal Clinical Diagnosis by Laboratory Methods. Philadelphia: W.B. Saunders Company.

INDEX

Boldface numbers indicate pages with figures.

ISBN 0-8138-2664-0

90000

9 780813 826646